DECODING

LONGEVITY

Ending Aging As We Know It

By

Bryant Villeponteau, Ph.D.

2

Copyright © 2013 by Bryant Villeponteau, Ph. D.

First Edition, December, 2013

Longevity Code
637 South Broadway
Boulder, CO 80305

Library of Congress Cataloging-in-Publication Data
LCCN: 2013921244
ISBN-13: 9781491211489

Preventive health books from *Longevity Code* are available at special bulk rates for private company special purchase or for educational distribution by nonprofit and professional organizations. Contact info@LongevityCode.com with specific request.

PUBLISHER'S NOTE: This book should not substitute for medical advice from your trained medical professional. Only your physician has the laboratory data on your current conditions and your medical history. Although the suggestions in this book are based on careful experimentation and recent scientific literature, individual differences can sometimes complicate any intervention. Neither the author nor the publisher takes responsibility for any possible consequences to individuals of the treatments and lifestyle changes recommended in this book.

Contents

4

Forward

> "Just remember when you are over the hill, you begin to pick up speed."

> **- Charles Schulz**

Have you ever wondered why aging occurs and how one might slow its progression? The aging research data in the last two decades offer many clues as to how we age and provide potential interventions to counteract the biochemical changes that lead to aging and human frailty. *Decoding Longevity* offers a full spectrum biological and genetic analysis of the aging process in layman's language. *Decoding Longevity* also discusses the exponential increases in technology that will likely lead to greatly expanded healthspan and longevity in the next 20 to 40 years.

The major aim of **Decoding Longevity** is to provide you with *Multipath Rejuvenation (MuR)* strategies that effectively slow multiple functional aspects of aging while preserving health and fitness well into your senior years. The key theme is staying alive and healthy using MuR strategies until the youth and healthspan revolutions are strongly accelerated by the stem cell and nano technologies in the coming decades.

With many fringe "experts" hyping growth hormone and other poorly researched antiaging strategies, scientists and the lay public have been properly skeptical of most life extension claims. However, the 21st Century provides real hope because of the longevity strides made since 1975 and especially the recent knowledge gained in the two decades since 1993. Indeed, science has made major progress in decoding many of the genetic and physiological causes of aging and the age-related diseases.

The popular idea that aging is simply the body 'wearing out' has been demonstrated to be largely myth. For example, a **single genetic alteration can extend worm lifespan 10 fold!** Aging, which was once thought to be the immutable and inevitable accumulation of damage, now appears to be surprisingly plastic. Moreover, some of the degenerative conditions once thought to be unavoidable consequences of aging are now believed to be preventable and may be reversible in many cases.

In response to this new knowledge, there have been a number of recent books on aging for both the academic and the lay reader. Unfortunately, the academic books are often difficult to read for the lay reader while most of the lay books over-hype selective aspects of the science and ignore other important developing areas.

The **first section of the Decoding Longevity** looks at the progress in the expansion of life expectancy in the 20th Century. The **second section** focuses on practical Multipath Rejuvenation (MuR) strategies that can significantly extend healthspan and youthful fitness in the present day. The **third section** looks in some detail at the last 25 years of aging research, while the **final section of the book** explores future developments that will provide powerful tools for extending healthspan and longevity in the next 20 to 40 years.

Science is a team effort and the field of aging has made remarkable progress based on the multipath attack by scientists in different fields of science using differing experimental systems. The fields of biochemistry, cell biology, evolutionary biology, developmental biology, neurobiology, genetics, stem cell biology, physiology, pharmacology, and even the information sciences have all played significant roles in our current understanding of aging. Different model biological systems (cultured human cells, human age-related diseases, yeast, worms, flies, rodents, primates, and human centenarians) have also played an essential role in advancing the field of aging research. The work with ***transgenic animals*** (animals whose genome has been altered by the transfer of genes from another species) has been particularly significant, as transgenic mutants have allowed us to determine the function of particular genes and their roles in aging. This has permitted the testing of many models of aging so as to focus on the critical common elements of biological aging. While other books have reported in greater detail on many of these experiments, none has focused on the principal drivers of the aging process with the single-minded goal of slowing or stopping its progression.

As a cautionary note, this book should not substitute for medical advice from your current medical doctors. We do, however, welcome information on your individual responses to the recommendations herein (see website **www.LongevityCode.com**). This will permit later editions of the book to incorporate the best treatments and lifestyle changes for extending healthspan.

Acknowledgements

While the views expressed here are largely my own, I am grateful to my many friends and colleagues in academia and industry whose research provided the basis for developing the longevity strategy outlined here. I give special thanks to Drs. Richard Adelman, Bruce Carlson, John Faulkner, Brant Fries, Ari Gafni, Jeffrey Halter, Richard Miller, and Duncan Steel from the *Institute of Gerontology* at the University of Michigan (see Medical School website http://www.med.umich.edu/geriatrics/research/IoG2.htm) for introducing me to the field of aging research when I was Assistant Professor of Biochemistry in the Institute. I also wish to thank the talented scientists that I interacted with in industry as Champion of Telomerase Therapy while at *Geron Corporation* (www.geron.com), as a member of the Scientific Advisory Boards of *Serra Sciences, LLC* (www.sierrasci.com) and the *Supercentenarian Research Foundation* (www.supercentenarian-research-foundation.org), and as Vice-President of Research and Development at *Genescient Inc. www.genescient.com* and at *Centagen Inc. www.centagen.com* : Drs. George Abraham, Richard Allsopp, William Andrews, Elizabeth Blackburn, Sylvia Bacchetti, Andrzej Bartke, Maria Blasco, Laura Briggs, Judith Campisi, Ed Chang, C.P Chiu, Robert Cockrell, Stephen Coles, James Curtsinger, Rita Effros, Calib Finch, Claudio Franceschi, Walter Funk, Fiderico Gaeta, Aubrey de Gray, Carol Greider, Lenard Hayflick, Cal Harley, David Harrison, Michal Jazwinski, Thomas Johnson, Pamela Larson, Serge Lichtsteiner, Tony Long, Edward Masoro, George Martin, Vincent Monnier, Laurence Mueller, James Murai, Mieczyslaw Piatyszek, Doros Platika, Michael Rose, G. Saretzki, Jerry Shay, James Watson,

Jan Vijg, Michael West, Tom von Zglinicki, Samuel Ward, and Woody Wright. I also give special thanks to Dr. Junli Feng (my wife), Dr. S Khalsa, Dr. George Martin, Carl Fowler, David Kekich, John M. Adams, and Debbie Nocita, who have reviewed the book before going to press.

1. Can Aging Be Slowed or Reversed?

> "The immortal Gods alone have neither age nor death! All other things Almighty Time disquiets."

- Oedipus by Sophocles

Whether you believe in an afterlife or not, no one likes the functional decline and chronic disorders that typically accompany aging. Age progressively weakens your fitness and health from a youthful 20 through the 50+ years when the aging process accelerates. The conventional wisdom has been that there is little that you can do about the declining health and fitness with age, so it is best to accept the inevitable and age gracefully. Before the 21st Century this conventional wisdom was largely correct and to believe otherwise was little more than wishful thinking. In the present day, this orthodox wisdom appears passé, as recent data strongly indicate that healthspan and life expectancy are far more changeable than anyone thought. Indeed, there are now many strategies that will make a significant difference in your rate of aging and you can even reverse some aspects. More importantly, our knowledge of how to enhance healthspan and longevity is increasing exponentially with new findings appearing weekly. Therefore, you don't have to passively accept aging and its associated functional decline in health and fitness. Instead, you can rationally choose the goal of retaining most aspects of health and fitness well into your senior years.

Even preventing the decline in health and fitness with advanced age will likely be possible in the not too distant future, as we will explore in the final chapter. Indeed, there are many examples of plants and animals where the annual mortality rate actually declines or stays the same with advancing age. For example, the Giant Sequoia trees shown on the book cover can live in excess of 3000 years, while the Bristle Cone Pine (**Pinus Longaeva**) can live some 5000 years. In the case of clonal trees, the **roots** of the "Pando" Aspen from the Fishlake National Park in Utah that have survived for an estimated 80,000 to 1,000,000 years without any signs of aging.

Pando Colony of a Single Male Aspen Tree

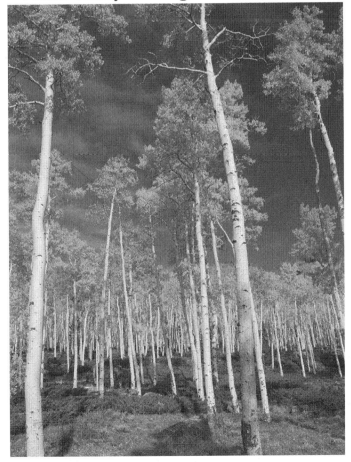

Very long and apparently ageless lifespans are not only found in plants. There are also animal species that do not appear to age and do not have observable increases in mortality rates with age (113). Some clams, hydras, lobsters, sea urchins, and sharks are examples of animal species with very low or nonexistent rates of fitness decline with age. The freshwater polyp Hydra is particularly well documented and basically shows that Hydra are essentially immortal (113). The existence of species with very low or zero rates of aging poses a real challenge for the damage or wear and tear theories of aging. But it fits well with the popular ***Evolutionary Theory of Aging***, which states that the lifespan of a species is dependent on environmental selection like other genetic traits of species.

In nature, the rate of aging appears to follow cues from the ecological niche that the species inhabits. For example, animals in dangerous environments typically have short lifespans (e.g. 1-3 years for small land rodents) while similar sized animals in safer environments removed from many predators (e.g. flying birds) often have much longer lifespans of 15 to 30 years. We will go into more detail on the Evolutionary Theory of Aging and what it means for the future of human aging in a later chapter.

What does the new research tell us about human aging and what can be done? You may have noticed that some people appear to age slower than others. What mix of genetics and lifestyle choices is responsible for their youthful looks? One fact that may be relevant here is that ***throughout recorded history the better educated have tended to live longer than the norm***. This book is dedicated to those who wish to educate themselves about how best to slow their aging rate and retain youthful fitness well into their senior years. My goal is to bring everyone up to date on the latest longevity data with the focus on doing what we can do now to survive until the 2040s. By 2050, the prediction is that we will have developed the technologies to preserve healthspan and fitness at advanced ages. Unfortunately, most in my generation (the baby boomers) and many in Generation X are unlikely to make it to this promised new era without significant effort on their part.

For nearly all of some 200 thousand years that modern humans have roamed earth, life expectancy has been distressingly short (about 30-35 years). If one did make it past 30, survivors in their 40s and 50s were considered old and most cases were old physiologically by today's standards. Of course, some hardy individuals in ancient times did live into their 70s, 80s, and even 90s, but this was rare. With high rates of childhood death, mean life expectancy in the US was only 49 years as recently as 1900. In the years 1901 to 2006 mean life expectancy had an unparalleled increase of about 28 years in the U.S. and other developed countries had similar increases. Indeed, the latter half of the 20th century was the first time in history that most individuals in wealthy countries had an expectation to live into their 70s and beyond.

Chapters 2 documents some of the data supporting this demographic explosion in the elderly population and *Chapter 3* explores many of the factors promoting humans reaching their current mean life expectancy of 77 to 81 years in the advanced countries.

Chapters 4 to 6 provide a practical guide to extending your personal longevity beyond the current U.S. life expectancy of 78 years and set a new personal goal of 100+ years. Surprisingly, the proposed preventive strategies for prolonging life will also extend youth, health, and fitness. Taking full advantage of the current antiaging technologies could add up to 25 years of healthy youth to your life. Most importantly, it may keep you alive and well enough that you could benefit from the major technological breakthroughs in medical and longevity research that will come along in the next 20 to 40 years culminating in much longer and perhaps indeterminate healthspans and lifespans.

Chapters 7 to 12 summarize the scientific data of the last 20 years on why and how we age. If scientific data bores you, these chapters of the book may be skipped. However, Chapters 7 to 12 are important for understanding both the rationale behind the practical recommendation found in Chapters 4 to 6 and the potential for radical changes in human lifespans by the 2040 to 2050 decade.

In *Chapter 13*, I forecast the future of the revolutionary technologies that will provide dramatic improvements in human healthspan and longevity. Indeed, these potential improvements in healthy life expectancy may even lead to **indefinite** healthspans by 2050. If one thinks that this is a wild and crazy statement, it is not. I describe the exponential growth in the relevant technologies that will power the revolutionary extension in human healthspan and lifespan.

Looking out 20 to 40 years, there are likely to be many bionic or nano technologies that will replace or dramatically enhance human capability, so as to compensate for or prevent losses due to aging and disease. The combination of both stem cell mediated organ regeneration and nanobot technologies will likely lead to bionic humans within the next 30 to 40 years, where health and fitness do not progressively decline with age. Note that people will still die via accidents, uncured diseases, and poor lifestyle choices, so this new technology does not promise immortality. Yet, the possibility of individuals living at a fully functioning youthful level and good health for well over a hundred years would be a seminal change in human existence that is more earth-shattering than any transformation in our long history as a species. In concert with others, I call this the **Longevity Escape Velocity**, where we gain one more year of healthspan and life expectancy for every year that we live.

Note that 30 to 40 years is not a very long period of time and many readers of this book could well be alive in 40 years. By following the recommendations in this book, you can greatly increase your chances of benefiting personally from this coming revolution. Are you up for the challenge? If so, then Decoding Longevity is a must read book for you and your loved ones.

2. A Century of Rising Life Expectancy

"Since 1950 the number of people celebrating their 100th birthdays has at least doubled each decade."

- Vaupel and Kistowski (74)

Summary: A Century of Rising Life Expectancy

Although increases in mean lifespan increased dramatically in the 20th century, true increases in human longevity post 60 years of age started around the 1970s and has been increasing incrementally ever since. As a result, people over 90 and 100 years of age are the fastest growing demography groups in the population in most developed countries of the world.

The will to live is clearly observed in all animal species. Indeed, avoiding death has long been a major preoccupation of most humans throughout recorded history. Nevertheless, before 1900, most humans who survived childhood lived a short life of 35 to 60 years. In many underdeveloped countries, this shortened adult lifespan remains the norm with most individuals dying prematurely from infectious diseases or from the inflammatory effects of chronic infections.

This traditional pattern changed dramatically for the economically advanced countries during the Twentieth Century. United States mean life expectancy was about 49 in

1900 and increased to about 77 years by 2000. ***That is a huge 57% increase in life expectancy in just 100 years.*** Moreover, life expectancy in the industrialized countries is still advancing: United States' life expectancy was over 78 years in 2007.

Increases in life expectancy do not mean that people actually had an extended life for those individuals lucky enough to make it past 60, and there is little evidence that maximum life span (about 120 years for humans) has changed. Before 1900, most people died prematurely from infectious diseases or later inflammatory complications of these diseases on cardiovascular health. The early 20th century gains in life expectancy mainly affected the percentage of people that lived to be 60, while life expectancy post 60 underwent little change before the 1950 to 1970 period. In this book, we will use ***longevity*** to designate the ***post 60 extended lifespan***, as this older population is clearly affected by aging and the age-related diseases.

The population over 60 years of age has been rising rapidly for nearly a century. For example, the percentage of the population over 65 in the United Kingdom increased from 6.1% in 1921 to 16.7% in 2001 and is estimated to become 20% in 2021 (Fig. 1). This is a 228% projected gain for the percentage of population over 65 in just 100 years!

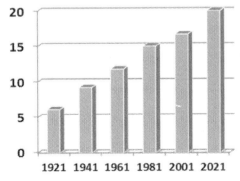

Fig. 1: Percentage of UK population over 65 years of age. Taken from UK census data from 1921 to 2001. Year 2021 is an estimate.

The percentage of population over 60 has also been projected to advance sharply though 2025 for the United States, Germany, Japan, and other major industrialized countries (US census bureau). The projected rates for 2025 of individuals over 60 are 24% in the US, 34% in Japan, and 33% in Germany. Much of the percentage increase in the over 60 population in the last 40 years can be explained by the marked decline in birthrates during the latter half of the 20th century, which drives a percentage increase in adults of all ages. For example, births in China dropped from 34 per thousand in 1969 to 16 per thousand in 1998 due to the stringent one-child policy followed by the Chinese government, and individuals over 60 are expected to rise from 10.9% in 2005 and to 20% in 2025.

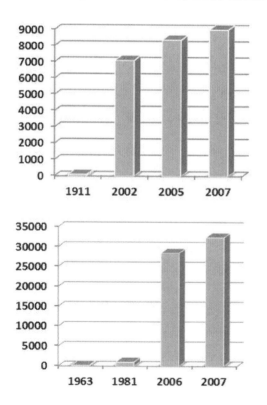

Fig. 2: Population of UK over 100 years of age. Taken from UK Census Data for years 1911, 2002, 2005, and 2007.

Fig. 3: Japan population over 100 years of age. Taken from Japan Census Data.

However, it is unlikely that all of the recent gains in the percentage of people over 60 are due to declines in birth rate. For example, the boom in centenarians in many developed countries is a strong indicator that longevity is rapidly advancing in the over 60 population apart from declines in birth rates. Figure 2 reveals a 70-fold increase in UK centenarians from 1911 to 2002 and the centenarian population continued to enlarge at a 4% annual rate after 2002, which is far higher than the rate of increase in total population. Japan has a longer life expectancy than the UK and its centenarian population is growing even faster. Figure 3 illustrates that Japanese centenarians increased 6.5-fold from 1963 to 1981 and then inflated 28-fold in the 25 year period from 1981 to 2006. As of 2006, the annual rate of centenarian growth in Japan is around 14%!

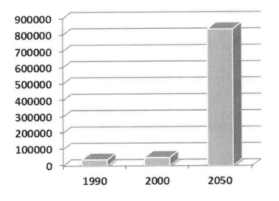

Fig. 4: United States population over 100 years of age. The years 1990 and 2000 were taken from U.S. Census Data. The projection for 2050 is from the International Longevity Center in New York.

In the case of the United States, the U.S. Census Bureau reported 37,306 centenarians in 1990 and 50,454 centenarians in 2001, which is a 35% increase in just 10 years. The number of U.S. centenarians is projected to increase to 834,000 people by 2050 (see Fig. 4), according to Dr. Robert Butler of the International Longevity Center in

New York City. ***Centenarians are thus the fastest growing segment of the U.S. population and the second fastest segment comprises those individuals over 85 years of age.*** The boom in centenarian populations and their projected rates of population growth are only possible because longevity rates are accelerating. Similar projections have been made for the other advanced countries of Europe and Asia, many with longevity increases higher than the US.

Although the common belief is that little or nothing can be done about aging, the above data and other recent research suggest that longevity is progressively rising in the population of advanced countries and shows no clear signs of reaching a limit (72-73). This raises many interesting questions: What are the specific factors generating increased longevity in advanced countries? Are there ways to promote longevity at a faster pace? Can individuals take specific actions now that will advance their own longevity and decrease their risks of age-related disease? Is there a natural limit to human longevity? The remainder of this book will attempt to answer these crucial questions.

The general goal of **Decoding Longevity** is to provide the reader with a personal guide to longevity based on current knowledge about the science of aging and about the prevention of age-related disease. To help in defining success in our longevity quest, we will identify short term metrics of longevity and health that serve as leading indicators of progress toward a longer and healthier life. Therefore, the emphasis in the book will be on identifying and reversing ***markers of functional aging***, so that one can readily measure progress toward better fitness and life extension.

In Chapters 4 to 6, I hope to motivate lifestyle changes to provide a longer and healthier life. Given the significant roles for diet, exercise, stress, supplements, and pharmaceuticals in aging, the book addresses specific ways to use the knowledge gained from recent scientific advances to significantly extend lifespan and healthspan. Personal motivation to change may also come from the realization that much more dramatic progress in life and youth extension is coming in the near future.

3. Causes of Rising Life Expectancy

"The Life history of the individual and his allotment of years is the resultant of inborn and environmental influences inextricably interwoven."

- Louis Dublin

Summary: Causes of Rising Life Expectancy

Improved nutrition, antibiotics, immunizations, lower inflammation, less smoking, control of lipids, and control of blood pressure have all contributed to longer mean life expectancy in the 20th Century and post-60 longevity in the last 40 years. Building on this foundation, the gains in longevity and healthspan can and will be exponentially bigger in the 21st Century.

Causes of Increased Life Expectancy in the 20th Century	Improved Sanitation	Improved Nutrition
	Antibiotics	Immunization
	Lower Inflammation	Less Smoking
	Lipid and BP Control	Regular Exercise

There was a remarkable increase in life expectancy during the twentieth century. While we may not have a complete understanding of human aging, we know a great deal more than we did twenty years ago. Most people think of aging as inborn and inevitable, but research suggests that aging is significantly affected by both genetics and the environment. Because human genetic evolutionary changes occur over hundreds and thousands of years, changes in the environment must account for nearly all of the increases in life expectancy over the last 100 years.

The early increases in twentieth century mean life expectancy are thought to be largely due to reduction in infectious disease. Most of the declines in morbidity and mortality likely come from improved sanitation and improved nutrition. Antibiotics and immunization also improved mean life expectancy in the years after World War II. All of these early changes in sanitation, nutrition, antibiotics, and immunization significantly reduced the risks of dying prematurely before age 60. The effects of these factors on the post 60 years are limited to the early inflammatory damage done to tissues and organs on exposure to infection at the early ages during the first part of the 20th century.

As we will examine later, inflammation is a major cause of age related disease and aging. Young survivors of major infections such as rheumatic fever often have accelerated cardiovascular disease and a shortened lifespan after age 60. Therefore, the survivors of the generations born before widespread use of antibiotics and immunization often suffered with high levels of inflammation from the infectious diseases that prematurely killed others in their generation 25 to 50 years earlier. Because of the long lag between initiation of inflammation and the appearance of age-related disease, clear improvement in the longevity rates for those over 60 did not appear in the US data until after 1970.

The causes of post 60 longevity increases since 1970 are still being studied, but clearly originate from many factors. First, the 25 to 50 year lag of inflammation damage from widespread exposure of early twentieth century generations to infectious diseases had dissipated by 1970. With the passing of the early generations exposed to inflammation from infectious diseases in their youths, the ability of improved nutrition, sanitation, antibiotics, and immunization to affect longevity in those over 60 became stronger in the developed countries in the years after 1950.

Allied with the decline in infectious disease, major lifestyle choices like ending smoking have played a major role in longevity. Smoking was in steep decline in the 1980 to 2000 period and fell by 27% in the US (40). Smoking is associated with increased mortality for many types of cancer, including a 13 to 23 fold increase in lung cancer risk, and significant increased risks for bladder, cervix, kidney, mouth, pancreas, and stomach cancers (60). Smoking is also a leading cause of cardiovascular disease with a 2 to 4 fold increased risk of heart disease (61) and a 2 fold increased risk of stroke (52). One way in which smoking is linked to general aging is that it causes reduced peripheral circulation by narrowing blood vessels (22). The decline in smoking in recent years in America and many European countries is likely one cause of increased longevity rates.

Other lifestyle choices like regular exercise and good diet are other predictors of mortality and thus may have been causes of the increased longevity. In the case of exercise, those humans who remain physically active have a substantial reduction in all-cause mortality and loss of motor function (7, 12, 35, 42, 48). Indeed, exercise is a major factor in increasing longevity for the subpopulation that is active. While many citizens in the US have become less active in recent years, the frequent advice to get more exercise in the last 30 years or so has led many to heed this guidance.

A healthy diet does help in preventing some of the age-related diseases and for more than 30 years the US government has recommended that individuals consume at least 5 servings of fruits and vegetables per day. The latest government guidelines recommend 5 to 13 servings per day (59) Those who follow this wise advice do have a lowered incidence of many chronic diseases (16, 37, 50). It is also true that the advent of cheap transportation by boat, rail, and truck in the early 20th century enabled the wide availability of fruit and vegetables year round. However, the average American currently eats 2 to 3 servings of fruits and vegetables per day and tends to consume too much processed sugary foods, so it is unclear how much diet has helped increase American longevity in recent years. This is not true for many European countries and Japan, which is likely to be one of the causes of their longer life expectancy.

Finally, one needs to look at the new drugs and medical techniques developed in the latter half of the twentieth century for treating cardiovascular disease, which remains the biggest cause of mortality and morbidity. The cardiovascular drugs that lower blood pressure and cholesterol are of greatest significance. For example, hypertension tends to increase markedly in those 50 years of age or older. Since the symptoms of hypertension are often silent and go undetected, many people are never treated for high blood pressure. Based on extensive study in the last 50 years, the role of hypertension in many chronic diseases has been recognized. More persistent screening of hypertensive patients and the existence of effective drugs has led to much better treatment of this all too common condition.

High cholesterol is another silent killer. The understanding of the role of cholesterol in promoting atherosclerosis led to close monitoring of cholesterol levels in individuals. This understanding also led to the development of effective anti-cholesterol drugs (statins) that have played an important role in the medicinal lowering of high cholesterol levels. However, statins can have serious side effects, so it is best to minimize the use of statins and rely mostly on dietary controls where possible.

Other modern medical advances such as the widespread use of organ transplants for those with severely damaged immune systems or heart, renal, liver, and lung failure have saved many from certain death. However, these technical advances have not yet made a significant impact on longevity. In many ways, modern medicine has perfected the science of delaying death from one cause, but often the price is prolonged pain and reduced function due to worsening from other diseases. Conversely, organ and cell replacement therapies based on the developing stem cell technologies should offer major longevity advancement as these techniques are perfected in the coming decades.

4. Anti-aging Dietary Program

"Ninety per cent of the diseases known to man are caused by cheap foodstuffs. You are what you eat."

- **The nutritionist Victor Lindlahr in 1923**

Summary: Anti-Aging Dietary Program

It may seem strange to start off a discussion of antiaging treatments by writing about diet. Can diet really be that important? The correct answer is that a good antiaging diet is currently the single best thing that you can alter to extend lifespan and healthspan. Indeed, the old saying that "you are what you eat" is a true statement in many respects.

Summing up all of the nutritional data that have been learned from the research studies comparing longevity, health, and various dietary regimens, there is a clear set of dietary principles that can be followed to maximize one's chances of a long healthy life while retaining the essential pleasures of eating.

1. Limit your intake of red meat, chicken, fish, and eggs to three or four 100 to 150 gram servings per week. Seafood is preferred over pork or chicken, which is better than beef or lamb. Dairy products like nonfat yogurt or low fat cheese are also allowed, but should be limited to one 6 to 8 once serving per day. Protein is critically important in the diet, but much of your daily protein intake should come from plant sources

like nuts and beans. Avoid the strict Vegan diet, as you may miss essential dietary factors.

2. Get 8 to 10 servings of fruit and vegetables per day. To make this easy and increase nutrient bioavailability, drink one or two smoothies per day with about 1/3 cup blueberries and 1/2 cup carrots and 1/3 cup broccoli or spinach and 3 prunes. Eat one apple and an orange per day along with a salad most days.

3. For the rest of your diet eat whole carbohydrates as much as possible. If you eat pasta or other carbohydrates with milled flour, then you should take supplements of various nutritional factors that are described in the supplement section. Also, if you eat milled flour products, it is very important to get extra bran such as 3 to 5 tablespoons of oat bran placed in heated water or smoothie for 1-2 minutes to expand. Yogurt or fruit can be added to add taste and texture to the bran before eating. But don't expect that eating 8 to 10 servings of fruit and vegetables gives you sufficient fiber if you are also eating significant amounts of processed grains and starches that lack fiber.

4. Minimize artificial sweeteners, salt, sugars, MSG, cookies, crackers, egg yolks, cakes, pastries, and junk food.

5. Avoid hydrogenated oils, fried foods, trans fat, and margarine. Minimize most vegetable oils that are rich in omega-6 fatty acid. Use canola or olive oils rather than the oils present in most other vegetable oils.

6. Try to get enough fiber and fermenting products to feed your intestinal microorganisms (microbiome). A healthy colon microbiome is essential for your health and longevity.

7. Healthy colon microorganisms should support one or more bowel movements per day without straining or excessive flatulence. If you do not have regular bowel movements, then fiber, "live culture" yogurt, and other micronutrients along with exercise should be added to support a healthy colon. The importance of human gut flora (the Microbiome) is detailed below.

Calorie Restriction (Reduced Food Intake)

Repeated studies beginning in the 1930s have used **Calorie Restriction (CR)** to generate enhanced mean and maximum longevity in many animal species. CR is a dietary regimen that reduces normal daily food intake from 20% to 50% of calories, which naturally extends lifespan by a factor of 10 to 60% depending on the species or conditions. CR has been demonstrated to work in rodents, flies, worms, yeast, dogs, and various fish species. The longest running CR experiment using Rhesus Monkeys has found health benefits and non-significant trends toward increases in median lifespan (as of November, 2012, 80% of the CR monkeys were still alive while 50% of controls had died). However, the monkey mean lifespan results to date have not reached statistical significance, which suggest that human benefits of CR on long lived primates might be more limited than observed in non-primate animals. Determinations of maximum monkey lifespans are still ongoing, so we do not know all the results of CR on primates. Unfortunately, the final results of this very long monkey CR experiment (23 years and still ongoing) may never be clear cut because of the small sample size and variable mortality. Yet the clear trend is that CR can slow aging in primates similarly, if less dramatically, to the case in lower animals.

Based on the above primate study and anecdotal human studies, it does appear likely that CR does have substantial benefits on age-related diseases. For example, human captives kept on starvation diets for many years in North Vietnam prisons have generally had fewer and less serious age related diseases than have comparable populations without this period of forced CR diet.

Aside from the issue of how efficacious CR is in humans, the problem is that CR is such a stressful diet that few people would consider it as a lifestyle choice. The common view is that eating is too much of a pleasure to go around hungry for most of your life just to be somewhat healthier and perhaps live a few years longer.

Fortunately, there is a little known technique to get most of the benefits of CR without being hungry or eating less food. It involves restricting animal protein rather than restricting total calories. Indeed, just restricting protein alone can generate 95% of the beneficial longevity results observed with full CR in *Drosophila*, which is a good model for human aging. Similar animal results with protein restriction have been observed in several other animal species.

In humans, protein restriction translates into eating low amounts of animal protein, as plant protein does not provide excessive amounts of the high quality protein that triggers faster aging. Indeed, the average lifespan of human vegetarians is reported to be several years longer than that found in meat eaters. And eating a high animal protein diet has been correlated with higher rates of cancer and heart disease. Therefore, the first recommendation is to eat less animal protein. ***While you do not have to be a strict vegetarian, try to eat animal proteins in moderate*** *amounts. Animal protein in the preferred form of fish or chicken should be consumed at the level of about three or four ounces 3 to 4 times per week.*

In trying to avoid excess animal protein, it is important to be moderate and avoid extremes. One extreme is to become a **vegan-vegetarian**, which means that you eat no animal products whatsoever and that you avoid dairy products as well. Most plant protein is deficient in certain required amino acids, so that a diet devoid of all high quality animal protein is often deficient in some of the required amino acids needed for body repair. That is the likely reason that vegans apparently have a somewhat shortened lifespan relative to those on a normal meat diet and a significantly lower lifespan than vegetarians who eat some dairy. While adults should avoid milk and most milk products, up to 8 ounces of plain nonfat yogurt per day is fine as is 1 to 3 ounces of cheese on occasion. The bacteria that transform milk into yogurt or cheese have health benefits beyond their high quality dairy proteins. When eating yogurt, and cheese, it is best to consume nonfat "live culture" yogurt and small portions of lower fat cheese. Almond milk may substitute for cow milk in cereal, recipes, or drinking.

Eat 8 to 10 Servings of Fruit and Vegetables Daily

Another very important dietary recommendation for health and longevity is to eat 8 to 10 servings of whole fruit and vegetables every day. Many research studies have demonstrated that fruit and vegetables prevent or delay age related disease. A favorable impact on aging is also inferred from the data showing longer lifespans in vegetarians and the data indicating that the processed foods in developed countries accelerates the onset of diabetes, cancer, and cardiovascular disease.

Of course, processed foods also contain excess added sugar and salt, which have been linked to diabetes, cancer, and heart disease. To make matters even worse, processed foods typically lack natural fiber, which permits sugars to be rapidly absorbed in the gut generating frequent glucose spikes in the bloodstream. The glucose spikes trigger insulin spikes that accelerate aging and disease.

The lack of fiber in processed foods further perturbs the intestines by slowing pass-through times and by enhancing the buildup of harmful bacteria. Both these factors lead to the chronic loss of healthy intestinal flora and mild to severe constipation, which helps to promote cancer, diabetes, and cardiovascular disease. A whole food diet promotes one or more bowel movements per day and this normal process of waste removal is required to keep your body fit and healthy.

OK, so you already knew that fruit and vegetables are good for you. But it is often difficult for most people to eat 8 or more servings of fruit and vegetables daily. Indeed, the average American only eats 2 to 3 servings of fruit and vegetables per day. Even if your own consumption is better than the average for Americans, how do you get 8 to 10 servings per day - particularly if you don't really like vegetables or enjoy many fruit choices? *Like the low protein diet substitution for CR, we need a dietary 'game changer' or the desirable goal of consuming more whole fruit and vegetables will typically fail for lack of compliance.*

The good news is that a good nutrition game changer is available! One can substitute *fruit and vegetable smoothies* to help you ingest the recommended daily quota of whole fruit and vegetables. Smoothies can be made from many different kinds of fruit and vegetables and make it far easier to get the desired 8 to 10 servings each day. Examples of good fruit components of the smoothie are: apples, blueberries, dried plums, 100% cherry juice extract, grapes, or strawberries. Examples of good vegetables to add are carrots, spinach, and broccoli. Surprisingly, none of these 3 vegetables detract from the taste and may even add sweetness. In contrast to home-made smoothies, nearly all the commercial smoothies are disasters with lots of sugar and even jam for fruit. Therefore, commercial smoothies should be largely avoided.

Having experimented with smoothies over a period of 20 years, I currently make 4 cups of the following smoothie for the whole family every morning:

Fruit and Vegetable Smoothie

Volume	Liquid, Fruit, or Vegetable
1 cup	Water
1 tablespoon	Lecithin
4	Dried Plums (Prunes)
3/4 cup	Frozen Blueberries
2/3 cup	Frozen Broccoli
1 cup	Cut and Peeled Carrots
1/4 cup	Cherry Juice Concentrate
3/4 cup	Almond Milk or Similar

The above mix of fruit and vegetables is blended in an ice-crushing Oster blender and then consumed within 10 minutes. The juice comes out rather thick and will gel into a solid if left longer than about 10 to 15 minutes. One glass of this smoothie every day is the equivalent of 5 or more servings of whole fruit and vegetables.

I normally make another smoothie for lunch that is much simpler. One version has 2/3 cups of water and a cut-up apple. A second version adds 1/2 cup spinach and one cup grapes. Other versions add a few grapes or strawberries to the apple. About one cup of the smoothie is put into a large 1.5 cup measuring glass and microwaved for 70 to 90 seconds. You can then add 4 heaping tablespoons of oat bran and mix. After a few minutes, about 3/4 cups of nonfat plain yogurt can be added and mixed before eating. This provides protein, whole fruit, and plenty of fiber.

Of course, the above juice recipes can be altered in many ways to account for your own taste and to provide variety. Indeed, when I started making smoothies many years ago, I used cut and peeled carrots and water, as regular stocks of freshly made commercial carrot juice were often not available. It was many years later that I improved on the carrot smoothies by adding many other kinds of fruits and vegetables. Smoothies can be changed endlessly to give variety.

I also caution that it is best to use whole fruit and vegetables for your smoothies. It is fine to use frozen blueberries and broccoli or spinach in the smoothie, as the quality of whole fruit and vegetables is not compromised by freezing. On the other hand, many commercial juices (whether canned or bottled) have been strained to remove fiber and they are inferior to smoothies made with whole fruit and vegetables. Also stay away from commercial "smoothies" that typically have commercial juice concentrates like apple or grape or even commercial jams as major ingredients. The best smoothie is the one you make yourself from whole fruit and vegetables and you should preferably drink it within 15 minutes of preparation.

Foods and Food Components to Minimize or Avoid

While most of the discussion above has focused on eating more fruit and vegetables, there are also some foods or food components that should be minimized or completely avoided. With all of the misinformation out there, it is valuable to look at the current evidence on this question.

One major example of a food component to be minimized is the **omega-6 fatty acids** found in most vegetable oils. While humans apparently evolved eating about a 1 to 1 ratio of omega-6 to **omega-3 fatty acids**, most people in the US and other western countries eat in excess of a 10 to 1 ratio. Many research studies have shown that high ratios of omega-6 to omega-3 fatty acids increase the risks of heart disease, cancer, rheumatoid arthritis, and other age related disease. Studies have further pointed to enhanced inflammation by high omega-6 to omega-3 consumption.

The best way to minimize risks from high omega-6 fatty acids is to avoid most plant oils from corn, palm, soybean, sunflower, and cottonseed. One advantage of canola (rapeseed) oil is that it has a higher omega-3 to omega-6 fatty acids ratios. Of course, the highest levels of omega-3 fatty acids are found in fish oil, so eating fish or taking fish oil supplements are other ways to increase your consumption of omega-3 fatty acids. But it is still important to minimize most of the common plant oils if you want to reduce the risks of inflammation and the chronic diseases.

Trans fat is another good example of a food component to avoid. Trans fat is commonly generated in the preparation of partially **hydrogenated vegetable oil,** which is mostly a man-made fat optimized for stability in the high-temperature cooking used to produce processed foods. Although rare in nature (e.g. < 4% in butter), trans fats are high in baking shortening (around 30%). Trans fats can also be found with most of the common poly-unsaturated plant oils. The polyunsaturated plant oils with the least potential for producing trans fats are olive and canola oils. Thus, olive and canola oils are the preferred polyunsaturated fats for cooking. However, the cooking oil with the least potential for trans-fat production is **extra virgin coconut oil**, which has beneficial medium chain saturated fatty acids and healthy antioxidant polyphenols.

Trans fats are known to raise LDL cholesterol and the inflammatory blood marker C-Reactive Protein (CRP), and believed to promote coronary heart disease. Inflammation inducing trans fats have also been associated with Alzheimer's disease, cancer, diabetes, liver dysfunction, infertility, and obesity. You can minimize exposure to the artery clogging trans fats by avoiding commercial cakes, pies, crackers, cookies, pastries, fried food, and junk food. When given a choice between butter and margarine, butter is a much better choice because it is lower in trans fat. The oils with the least trans fats are coconut, olive, and canola in that order. Any of these three oils is a better choice than the unhealthy trans-fat oils like corn, palm, or soybean oils.

Another food component to minimize is sodium glutamate (aka MSG, Ac'cent, Aji-No-Moto, and Vetsin). MSG is a non-essential amino acid used for more than a 100 years by food manufactures as a potent flavor or taste enhancer for meat, vegetables, marinades, sauces, and soups. MSG also improves the taste of low sodium foods, so search for it in foods touted as low salt. The safety of MSG has been reviewed many times, but with the exception of MSG-sensitive individuals, the studies have failed to observe adverse effects of MSG on chronic illnesses at normal doses. However, given that glutamates are brain-active neurotransmitters that cause hyperactivity or headaches in some individuals, it is best to curtail the consumption of foods containing MSG.

Artificial sweeteners are other taste enhancers that are best curtailed or avoided. Aspartame, sucralose, neotame, acesulfame, saccharin and stevia are the artificial sweeteners that are approved for use by the FDA as food additives to replace sugar. All of these sugar substitutes are synthesized chemicals with the exception of stevia. Even extensive animal and human studies have not quelled all of the safety questions on the use of these artificial sweeteners. For example, the safety of the most popular sweetener aspartame (Nutrasweet) has been extensively studied in animals and humans and is now approved for use in almost every country. While there are a few people that may be allergic, headaches are the most common symptom reported with aspartame. Since we do not know the effects of lifetime consumption, it is best to minimize the use of synthetic sweeteners in favor of natural sweeteners like stevia. Stevia, along with sorbitol and xylitol, are alternative natural sugar substitutes that are apparently safer and even have some positive benefits.

Any discussion of artificial sweeteners is incomplete without discussing the most prevalent food additives: cane sugar and fructose. These natural sugars have been added to drinks and most processed foods to enhance taste. Sugar and fructose are ubiquitous empty calorie food additives that strongly promote obesity and many health problems. Thus, minimizing your consumption of sugar is a very important goal for longevity. But the "sugar high" is quite addictive and most processed foods add sugar, so stopping all sugar consumption is nearly impossible in the US. That is one reason why there is such a huge market for the synthetic sweeteners. Shifting to stevia as an added sweetener is optimal in these cases.

Finally, there is the issue of animal protein, which is a good example of a food group to be reduced as we discussed above. My basic recommendation is to limit animal protein to 3 or 4 ounces of fish, chicken, or pork for 3 or 4 days of the week. Wild-caught fish and free-range chickens are best. Hot dogs, hamburgers, and most luncheon meats should be avoided, as these products typically have potentially harmful food preservatives such as sodium nitrite.

In the case of dairy products, adults over 20 should avoid milk or ice cream. Plain nonfat yogurt is fine, as the milk casein protein has been extensively processed by the lacto bacteria in the yogurt, which provides beneficial bacteria for your colon. Fermented cheeses should be consumed in limited amounts as a condiment to add taste or texture to food. Egg whites are fine in limited amounts, but avoid egg yolks unless the hens are free-range and fed with omega-3 oils.

General Overall Diet

We should also address the overall diet as it relates to the potential for an extended life of fitness and health. This is a huge subject with new diet books coming out all the time. There are many theories on the best diet and the field of nutrition is always coming out with new things. But if we limit ourselves to what is now known to promote health and longevity, then we can best describe an overall diet that can succeed in making a permanent change in your lifestyle to keep you healthy and fit without destroying the joy of eating as one of life's essential pleasures.

Perhaps the best way to proceed is to give an historic perspective on the progression of dietary thought as differing diets became the subject of serious research and discussion over the last 50 years. Note that my focus is on dietary changes that yield better overall health and longer life, rather than on the popular area of weight loss diets. As it turns out, the best diet for health and longevity is likely a diet that will also keep you slim.

In the 1960s, many of the ideas on diet that dominate today had already appeared. For example, vegetarians (no meat) and vegans (no meat or eggs or dairy products) were already well represented in many places. The family members of one of my best friends were vegetarians that believed in drinking carrot and cabbage juice along with large salads and vitamin supplements. They had many popular books on juice regimens, which claimed that most human diseases could be prevented or cured by drinking fresh juices. Of course, the preferred method for preparing juice in the 1960s was a $2000 hydraulic press juicer, where the juice pulp was thrown away. Hydraulic pressed juice is much thicker than standard commercial juices, as it had more fiber and other nutritional factors than did the highly filtered commercial juices.

Of course, in the late 60s, the vegetarian lifestyle with its focus on freshly made vegetable juices was not the expert opinion of professionals on what was then thought to be ideal nutrition. Indeed, this was before the US government's recommendation that we eat 4 or 5 servings of fresh fruit and vegetables daily, which was recently revised to 8 to 9 serving per day.

Back in the early 70s, I was initially skeptical of many of the vegetable juice claims, but realized that even if only a small fraction of the claims for juice therapy were true, it would be well worth the effort to make juice therapy a part of one's lifestyle. Not wanting the expense or messy work required with a juice extractor, I took the easy route of buying commercial carrot juice one or more times a week.

As more scientific evidence verified that eating whole fruit and vegetables lowered disease risks, I started trying to eat more of that type of food rather than grains or meat. My progression to a fruit and vegetable diet was enhanced in the early 1980s by the arrival of the **Pritikin diet**. Nathan Pritikin's diet book entitled "The Pritikin Program for Diet and Exercise" focused on a low fat diet of minimally processed fruit, vegetables, beans, potatoes, yams, whole grains, lean meat, and seafood. Several studies have shown that the Pritikin diet lowers cholesterol, C-reactive protein, blood sugar, blood pressure, and excess weight. The risks of heart disease and diabetes are also greatly reduced with the Pritikin diet.

The **Ornish diet** was another similar low fat dietary approach that appeared in the 1980s. It promotes whole food and a plant based diet that permits occasional animal protein. Dr. Dean Ornish wrote best-selling books and authored major scientific studies showing the benefits of his diet and other lifestyle changes in slowing, stopping, and even reversing the progression of coronary artery disease. Other medical doctors like Caldwell Esselstyn have demonstrated similar positive benefits in cardiac patients.

The **South Beach diet** is worth mentioning as an extension of the Pritikin and Ornish diets. The South Beach diet was designed by the cardiologist Arthur Agatston in the early 2000s. Agatston found that many of his patients indicated that the low fat diets of Pritikin and Ornish were difficult to follow in practice, so he set out to make modifications that would promote higher compliance rates for a healthy diet that his heart patients could stay on long term. Since many on a low fat diet ended up compensating for the low fat by eating more simple carbohydrates that often led to recurring hunger cycles, Dr. Agatston added satisfying fatty foods like nuts, lean meat, and eggs to the South Beach diet. While Dr. Agaston permits more animal protein and fat than does Pritikin or Ornish, Dr. Agaston rejected the alternative high protein, high fat, and low-carbohydrate **Atkin's diet** as not sufficiently beneficial or healthy.

The South Beach diet sets up *two simple dietary principles to guide food selection: 1) Substitute 'good carbs' (low glycemic carbohydrates that do not induce insulin spikes) for 'bad carbs' (empty calories that induce high blood glucose and insulin spikes); 2) Substitute 'good fats' (unsaturated fats and omega-3 fats) for 'bad fats' (trans-fats and saturated fats)*. Clinical studies published in 2004 and 2005 studies have shown favorable health results for the South Beach Diet. The end goal of the South Beach diet is higher nutritional compliance by individuals to a diet with a healthy outcome.

The **Mediterranean diet** is still another great diet that is based on the traditional diet found in southern Italy and France, Greece, Span, and Morocco. The Mediterranean diet is higher in fat and protein than the Pritikin or Ornish diets and permits dairy products (mainly cheese and yogurt) with some fish, chicken, red meat, and wine, even though the bulk of the diet consists of whole fruit, vegetables, grains, and olive oil. While the Mediterranean diet has obviously been around for centuries, it only gained widespread recognition in the US in the 1990s when the Seven Countries Study reported favorable health benefits and low rates of cardiovascular disease and overall mortality for populations on the Mediterranean diet. Note that the Mediterranean diet has many similarities to the South Beach diet and there are even vegetarian variations on the South Beach diet that are high in carbohydrates.

The **Paleolithic diet** is one final diet that is worth mentioning based on its claimed scientific basis in human evolution. The Paleolithic diet (aka **Caveman** or **Hunter-Gatherer** or **Paleo diet**) consists of fish, free-range animal meat, fruit, vegetables, roots, and nuts, but excludes grains, legumes, processed oils, or processed sugar. This diet is promoted by some evolutionary biologists, who claim that we evolved as a species on this diet and have had insufficient time to adapt genetically to the grains, dairy products, and other foods prevalent in the post-agricultural revolution of about 10,000 years ago.

The Paleo diet has been criticized by dietitians (for the emphasis on high animal protein intake and the avoidance of grain products), anthropologists (for the claims that ancient societies did not suffer from "diseases of civilization" and that pre-agricultural man did not eat grains), and biologists (who question the evolutionary logic). Indeed, recent rankings by one 2012 group of 24 experts rated the Paleo diet the lowest of the 24 diets that they rated based on health, weight-loss, and ease of following. Nevertheless, the claims that most indigenous peoples today do not eat processed food and are generally free from many degenerative diseases do appear generally accurate, so some aspects of the Paleo diet are likely true. My conclusion is that the Paleo diet is on strong ground in recommending whole foods and the avoidance of processed grain products stripped of fiber and nutrients that are so prevalent in developed countries. As a complete diet though, the Mediterranean or South Beach diets are easier to follow and likely better than Paleo diets that are hypothesized to be eaten in pre-agriculture times based on incomplete data. The Paleo focus on high meat intake is particularly problematic. Also, the Paleo diet's appeal to avoid grain products is not supported by experimental data with the exception of high gluten grains, which a few individuals are unable to process for lack of properly functioning intestinal enzymes.

The Effects of Diet on Human Gut Flora (Microbiome)

No discussion of the effects of diet on aging is complete without emphasizing the importance of your intestinal microorganisms (the **microbiome**). A healthy colon is a key factor in health and is based on maintaining a diverse complement of healthy gut bacteria. Unhealthy gut microorganisms can render the colon more permeable to endotoxins and inflammation, speed glucose uptake to promote diabetes, and greatly slow progression of fecal matter through the intestines promoting constipation and increased adipose cell growth.

Fortunately, retaining a healthy colon microbiome is largely a healthy side effect of consuming a whole food diet with ample non-digestible fiber and fermented foods such as yogurt or kefir. A healthy diet for your gut flora should include **resistant starches** (e.g. beans, oats, and bananas), **soluble fiber** (e.g. onions, root vegetables, and nuts), and **insoluble fiber** (e.g. whole grains and oat bran). To get a variety of beneficial bacteria, eat plain yogurt or Kefirs with live cultures. Many types of cheese are also good sources of healthy gut bacteria: examples include goat cheese, parmesan, cheddar, provolone, feta, Gouda, and gruyere. Of course, you should monitor your cheese intake, as a little can promote valuable gut flora, while overdosing could promote unhealthy blood cholesterol levels and excessive calorie intake. Finally, there are fermented vegetables like kimchee and sauerkraut. Pickled foods are also fermented, but are best avoided.

So how do you know if your microbiome is functioning well? If you are eating a healthy whole food diet with adequate fiber and live bacteria, you are probably on the right track. But you need to remember that antibiotics (present in some meat or milk products) and some processed foods can kill off your healthy gut flora. If that happens, a healthy gut flora can be restored by going back on the whole foods and fermented products. Positive indications of a healthy colon are frequent and easy bowel movements and the absence of gas or intestinal pain.

Note that frequent exercise also promotes regular bowel movements, while a sedentary lifestyle can readily lead to sluggish bowel movements and the growth of unhealthy gut flora.

An Enjoyable and Healthy Longevity Diet

If you follow the above low inflammation, whole food, and low protein diet, you will greatly lower your risks for the age-related diseases. The all-important circulatory system (arteries, capillaries, and veins) will be better preserved with age, as the buildup of arterial plaque should decrease rather than increase. The age-related thinning out of the capillary structure that delivers blood glucose and oxygen to your vital organs will be slowed.

The above diet should also help prevent the typical buildup of inflammation, LDL cholesterol, oxidized-LDL, and insulin resistance with age, which are all major factors in many degenerative diseases. Coupled with moderate exercise, the anti-aging diet will slow or avert the typical loss of bone and muscle with age. Even the risk of cancer will be reduced by: promoting faster turnover of damaged tissues that are likely to become cancerous, inhibiting cancer cell growth with plant based flavonoids, promoting optimal gut flora that produce a healthy colon, and strengthening the immune response to cancer cells.

Finally, the anti-aging diet should help slow the loss of hearing, taste, touch, smell, and vision that gradually progress as we age. The 5 senses are an important part of being alive and one of the main reasons that youth is valued. The other benefits of youth are energy, the capacity for deep sleep, mobility, and freedom from chronic pain. The anti-aging diet can help in all these areas as well and is an absolutely essential component of any strategy to preserve health and vitality as we age.

5. Anti-aging Exercise Program

"Lack of activity destroys the good condition of every human being, while movement and methodical physical exercise save it and preserve it."

- The Greek philosopher Plato

Summary: Anti-Aging Exercise Program

As indicated by the above quote by the famous Greek philosopher Plato from around 340 BC, it has been known for a very long time that lack of activity is not compatible with health and wellbeing. Yet, everyone knows that most of us tend to be less active with age. How do we change this dynamic and get the exercise that is optimal for health and longevity?

1. Activity and exercise are essential for most aspects of health and vitality with longevity as an important side effect.
2. All movement activities count as beneficial (even housework and walking), so no one should argue that they don't have the time or the discipline to be active.
3. Aim for 20 to 40 minutes of endurance training per day with your heart rate raised over 110 beats per minute, which may include brisk walks, run-walks, biking, tennis, swimming, gardening, basketball, etc.
4. Stretch for 5 to 10 minutes 3 or 4 times a week.

5. Do 15 minutes of high repetition (20+) resistance training for 3 or 4 times a week using barbells, dumbbells, exercise wheels, and/or body weight (e.g. pushups, stomach crunches, and leg raises).
6. Avoid long hard workouts or races (60 minutes or more) where your heart rate is near its maximum and you are overly tired, frequently injured, or stressed out.
7. If you are sitting down inactive for 2-4 hours, perform 2-5 min of exercise to get your circulation going again.

The Benefits of Exercise and the Costs of Inactivity

Keeping active is universally recognized as good for your body. There are many benefits of keeping active and personal costs to an inactive lifestyle. The main benefits of exercise are:

1. Promotes longevity and lowers risks of disease.
2. Boosts energy and zest for life.
3. Improves brain function and mood.
4. Reduces weight.
5. Promotes better sleep.
6. Improves sex life.
7. Stimulates the immune system.
8. Lowers injury rates in bones, muscles, and joints.
9. Keeps you fit for activities with friends and family.
10. Provides fun and enjoyable activities.

A positive correlation of longevity with moderate exercise has been proven in many studies with many animal species. Likewise, human studies have shown that moderate exercise greatly improves circulation and heart function. For example, moderate exercise lowers resting pulse rate and blood pressure. Indeed, for some hypertensive people moderate exercise can effectively bring down blood pressure into the normal range of 120/80 mm Hg or lower. Blood sugar is also much better controlled with exercise as are LDL cholesterol and the triglycerides.

More energy may seem like an unlikely benefit of exercise, as inactivity makes everything physical seem like a big effort. But *regular moderate activity actually makes you feel less lazy and more willing to do something active*. Most importantly, regular exercise boosts bone growth, a more efficient circulatory system, better endurance (oxygen capacity goes up), heart function, and muscle strength. Life just gets a whole lot easier with regular exercise.

Movement and stressful activity are essential for bone growth. The lack of stressful activity on bone is the reason for bone loss in astronauts in zero gravity space, so expect excessive bone loss if you spend your whole day sitting or lying down.

In the case of the circulatory system, *small capillaries that feed all the organ systems typically decline significantly with age causing the buildup of fat cells, fibrosis, and cell aging. Exercise slows all of these processes down and sometimes can even reverse them by promoting capillary growth.*

The decline in muscle strength with age is often thought to be intrinsic, but even people in their 70s and 80s can build muscle if they regularly work out. Of course, if your muscles have grown flabby and fibrotic from 5+ years of disuse, then growing new muscle will be much more challenging and you will have to proceed slowly and with great care to avoid injury.

It also may surprise some people that exercise improves neural function, memory loss, and mood, but many studies have shown this to be true. Memory, muscle coordination, and reflexes all tend to decline with aging and inactivity. *Exercise increases brain circulation and neural factors that promote neural stem cells, memory, better muscle coordination, and faster reflexes.* There is also an improvement in mood after exercise, which comes from several factors including the stimulation of chemicals in the brain that leave you feeling more relaxed and happy.

If you want to lose weight, then exercise is an essential component of successful weight loss. First, moderate exercise depresses appetite, so you tend to eat less. Second, exercise revs up your metabolism so as to burn extra calories. Third, exercise builds muscle and reduces fat to make movement easier and less taxing on your joints and ligaments.

There are many positive effects of exercise on preventing disease. One of the most important disease preventing effects of exercise is to strengthen the immune system. For example, the number of disease fighting T cells can double with regular exercise, which provides a stronger defense against both bacterial and viral diseases. As the immune system weakens with age, chronic infections become more common and persistent, which is a strong promoter of high levels of chronic inflammation. And chronic inflammation is a basic cause of many age related diseases such as arthritis, cancer, dementia, and heart disease.

Physical intimacy is another area that is helped by more exercise. With age many people feel ashamed to bare their pale and flabby flesh, so adding muscle and definition in place of flab can really help your self-esteem. But regular exercise also enhances arousal and sexual function in both women and men. Equally priceless is that fertility is also increased by regular exercise.

Most people have trouble sleeping well as they age. Sleep problems can vary from sleep apnea to problems in falling asleep or staying asleep. Few things are more frustrating than waking up in the middle of the night and not being able to fall back asleep. Regular exercise generally helps with these common sleep problems and often reduces the number of hours of sleep needed.

Even with all the clear benefits to exercise, most people have problems following an effective exercise regime. Some claim they are too busy. But a highly effective exercise program would only take about 20 to 30 minutes a day (see below) and that could be 'paid for' time wise by needing less sleep. Indeed, many of the busiest people in the world take the time to exercise regularly, as exercise also clears the mind and makes you more productive.

Even if you feel you cannot spend 30 minutes per day for formal exercise, everyone can afford 15 to 20 minutes. Recognize that just 15 minutes per day is far better for your health than doing nothing. Also note that **walking is better than standing still, which is better than sitting, which is better than lying down. So try to keep as active as possible throughout the day.**

One last fact is important to know. Any exercise that is vigorous enough to generate sweat and heavy breathing (oxygen deficit) will 'reset' your whole metabolism. Your body typically responds to exercise stress, oxygen deficit, and any induced pain with the induction of various systemic factors and hormones. The induced factors and hormones slowly decay over a 24 hour period and continue to provide health and mood benefits long after the exercise is completed.

To many people, exercise can be painful or at least uncomfortable. The old saying "no pain, no gain" has some truth to it when referring to vigorous exercise. ***But for 20 to 30 minutes of discomfort, you are rewarded by many hours of elevated mood due to the increased endorphin levels in the brain.*** Endorphins are nature's morphine that is induced during injury or stress. Drug addicts who take narcotics depress their natural endorphin levels leading to withdrawal pains when the narcotic is finally excreted. Strenuous exercise inverts this process by increasing the level of natural endorphins to give a natural high long after the discomforting activity has ceased.

In the longer term, exercise may not get easier, but you get stronger, healthier, and feel less pain throughout the day. In my view, that is the tradeoff (short term discomfort for longer term relief from chronic pain and feel-good highs) that makes strenuous workouts worth all the effort. But for those that can't do strenuous exercise, even mild or casual exercise is still helpful.

Physical Activity for Health and Longevity

There are innumerable types of physical activities that humans have engaged in and a more limited set of reasons for exercising. Most people engage in physical activity for fun, weight loss, health, or enhanced fitness. If our goal is longevity and health, then the question is what types of activities are optimal for these goals and how much exercise is desirable for optimal longevity and health. Fortunately, research in both animals and humans gives good answers to these questions.

To maximize health and longevity, it is best to do about 20 to 40 minutes of vigorous exercise every day. The 20 to 40 minutes of activity should ideally include both aerobic and non-aerobic exercises so all muscle groups are exercised. If major muscle groups are left out, then this increases your risks of injury when the unexercised muscle group is suddenly called into action by one of your movements and is damaged due to unaccustomed activity.

Below I will describe an exercise program that attempts to meet these ideal exercise goals while minimizing time and effort. But before going into the details of an example of a specific exercise regime, I will describe three basic activity groups for designing your own custom exercise program for health and longevity.

As the first activity group, **endurance training** (aka **aerobic exercise**) strengthens your heart and helps (with the right diet) keep your arteries elastic and free of plaque. Endurance training also reduces body fat, cholesterol, blood sugar, and blood pressure. Mood, reflexes, coordination, memory, and the quality of sleep are all promoted by endurance exercise.

Examples of endurance exercises are biking, running swimming, fast walking, hiking, and any competitive sport or gym activity that gets your heart rate elevated above 110 beats per minute for 20 minutes or more. A minimum of 20 minutes per day four to seven days per week should be expended on endurance activities.

But don't overdo it, as frequent strenuous endurance activities lasting more than 40 minutes may be detrimental and promote aging. The reason is that strenuous activity gives sufficient benefits within 20 minutes with most endurance exercises, while the negatives side effects (high oxidative stress levels, joint, foot, and muscle injuries) of the strenuous activity start to multiply with longer times of 60 to 180 minutes per day. Moreover, while marathons and triathlons can make you very fit in the short run, 10 to 30 years of activity at this high performance level can increase your rate of aging. Multiple runs of 2 to 3 miles some 3 or 4 days per week are sufficient for maximum longevity benefits without undue injury and stress if proper diet and stretching are followed.

Another way to overdo exercise is to routinely perform at extreme levels for 10 to 30 minutes or more. For example, if you run at a fast constant rate for 20 to 30 minutes or more, you may be overdoing it if your heart rate is typically over the recommended maximum heart rate calculated by the formula 220 beats per minute minus your age. However, short sprint runs are good for you if completed within 100 seconds or less. Many animals in nature (e.g. lions and tigers) hunt other animals by sprinting for short distances with sprint times of 20 to 60 seconds to catch their prey. Copying nature, it is wise to insert 2 or 3 short maximum speed sprints of 30 to 90 seconds into a longer more leisurely walk or run.

If you are like most people and prefer more leisurely endurance activities, then take brisk 20 to 40 minute walks at least 3 or 4 times per week. It is normally best to combine some of your walks with 2 to 3 short 40 to 60 second sprints to exercise a different set of muscles and reset your cardiovascular system. This strategy is called *interval training*, which is well documented to be very efficient for building fitness and endurance.

A second activity group is *resistance training*, which can reverse muscle loss and helps maintain muscle tone into late old age. Resistance training is not the only path to maintaining muscle mass as you age, but it takes the least time and is the most efficient activity for maintaining muscle mass. Examples of resistance training are the use of free weights, weight machines, push-ups, sit-ups, pull-ups, and leg raises.

The goal is to exercise all muscle groups, especially in the arms, abdominal core, and back. One can also use resistance training to exercise your legs, but this is not necessary if you run, dance, walk, or play a competitive sport where you get good leg workouts. It is best to do resistance training sessions of 15 to 20 minutes some 3 or 4 times per week. Also, it is important to do at least 20 repetitions of any resistance exercise and work up to 40 to 100 repetitions, as you are less likely to injure yourself with low reps and high reps give you some endurance training as well. Resistance training should also not be the only exercise that you do in a workout. It is best combined with 20 minutes of endurance exercise and a few minutes stretching in the same workout.

The last activity group is ***stretching***, which is essential to keep you limber and free of injury in your other workout and daily activities. Stretching also improves athletic performance. The goal is to stretch all limbs and especially the neck and back. For example, a great lower back stretch is the Superman (see exercise video for detailed visuals at http://www.bodybuilding.com/exercises/detail/view/name /superman), which can come in several variations such as: arms out front as shown, arms behind head, or arms strait back. Another important stretch is to sit on the floor with your legs split and stretch your arms out to your left and then right foot. Then twist around to face toward your back. Stomach crunches and leg raises are great combinations for both stretching and resistance training.

An Exercise Program for Health and Longevity

Below I give a specific exercise program that is an example of what has worked as a very efficient program to maintain high levels of fitness and health. The weekly schedule is as follows:

1. **Sunday** – 20 minutes of stretch/resistance training followed by a 50 minute brisk walk.
2. **Monday** - 20 minutes of stretch/resistance training followed by a 20 minute walk/run.
3. **Tuesday** – 30 minute run at various effort levels.
4. **Wednesday** - 20 minutes of stretch/resistance training followed by a 22 minute walk/run.
5. **Thursday** – 30 minute run at various effort levels.
6. **Friday** - 20 minutes of stretch/resistance training followed by a 20 minute walk/run.
7. **Saturday** – 30 minute run at various effort levels.

In the above exercise program, 50 minutes of biking, tennis, basketball, swimming, or brisk walking can be substituted for the 30 minute run. In substituting swimming, walking, or biking for running it is best to vary the speed of the exercise, so that you have several short 40 to 60 second spurts at maximal activity levels. The recommended time would generally be higher in the case of less stressful exercise, because the effort is much lower. For example, a 30 minute swim is the rough equivalent of a 30 minute run or jog. However, walking or biking typically takes longer (40 to 50 minutes) for maximum benefit. In comparing different types of exercise, one can use the Aerobics Point System developed by Dr. Kenneth Cooper that calculates the intensity and duration of differing types of activities (e.g. see page 9 to 11 of the ***Navy Personal Trainer Program*** PDF at http://www.northwestern.edu/nrotc/docs/NavPersTrainPro g.pdf). The goal is to get 30 points or more per week.

If you do the maximum in the above weekly exercise program using running, run-walks, and the other the stretch/resistant training recommended, you would be getting roughly 100 points on the Cooper Aerobics Point System, which is the level at which athletes perform. It is not recommended to go higher than 100 points per week and you can be quite healthy getting just 30 to 50 points per week. Indeed, Dr. Cooper's studies have shown that most of the best health benefits occur with just 30 points, which can be obtained by working out only 3 days per week. However, *it is still important to get a mix of endurance, resistance and stretch activities if you want to maximize your health and prevent activity related injuries.*

Longevity Stretch and Resistance Training Program

The Longevity Stretch and Resistance Training Program as described below is a high performance exercise and stretching program that should be started at a very low level for each exercise if you have not exercised your back and abdominal muscles for a year or more. Even the minimum of 15 repetitions may be too much if you are like most people and failed to exercise most of your abdominal and back muscles as you have matured. Even bones and cartilage are weakened by years of disuse or chronic inflammation, so *you have to take any new back and stomach exercises very slowly at first if you want to avoid injury*. However, if you begin with low repetitions and add 1 or 2 reps per week over a period of 25 to 50 weeks, you should be able to improve greatly without major injuries.

A video of my favored 10 to 25 minute stretch/resistance training program is available under "Longevity Training" on **You Tube**: see the stretch/resistance video at https://www.youtube.com/watch?v=8EWqJtfRnw0. A verbal description is as follows:

1. **Superman Back Stretch** where you lay flat on your stomach, put your arms behind your head, and arch up your feet and head simultaneously. Repeat 15 to 40 times. Then put your arm straight back and arch up your feet and head simultaneously. Repeat 15 to 40 times. Then put your arms forward and arch up your feet, head, and arms simultaneously. Repeat 15 to 40 times. Then put your hand behind your head again and arch up your feet and head simultaneously. Repeat 15 to 40 times.

2. Do 15 to 50 **pushups** in less than 2 minutes. Rest a minute.

3. Lie on back and do 20 to 100 **stomach crunches**. Follow with 20 to 100 elbow to opposite leg crossover stomach crunches. Follow with 20 to 100 perpendicular leg raises with back flat on floor. Follow with 20 to 100 leg kicks lying flat on floor. Follow with back arch with feet and hands touching floor and hold for 3 seconds.

4. **Stretches:** Sit up and place legs in front of you. Try to touch your toes and hold for 3 seconds. Fold left leg to touch right thigh and then try to touch right toes with both hands stretched out and then repeat with right leg. Then cross left leg over right leg and turn head to view toward your rear. Repeat with left leg. Put legs out straight and touch toes with both hands. Then put

both legs split in front of you and touch both hands to feet.

5. ***Exercise Wheel:*** Get on your hands and knees and grab an Exercise Wheel for abs and push the exercise wheel forward in front of you some 20 to 100 times. You should go out extra far with the last 10 to 20 wheel pushes forcing elbows to almost touch the floor to fully extend back and arms.

6. ***Dumbbells:*** Using a pair of dumbbells of 5 to 20 pounds stand straight up and curl the dumbbells toward your chest. Repeat with a swinging motion 15 to 60 times. Follow with lifting the dumbbells to your shoulder and then lift over your head. Repeat the shoulder dumbbell lifts 10 to 40 times.

Once mastered, the above 6-step stretch/resistance training regimen provides the flexibility and strength to avoid injury in everyday activities and sports. It is designed to combine resistance training and stretching to all muscle groups in the upper torso while also providing significant endurance training for the back, stomach, and arms. Yet it does not take much time or risk injury using heavy weights and low reps. Avoid very heavy weight lifting in which the maximum number of reps is 12 or less. If your goal is health and longevity, then 15 or more replications of a resistance exercise in a single set is the proper goal, not low reps and heavy weights. If big muscles are your priority, then heavy weights are essential, but the above workout will help prevent injury with the heavy weights.

This set of resistance/stretch exercises should be followed by a brisk walk or walk/run of 20 to 40 minutes. Of course, other aerobic activities such as swimming, biking, or tennis could substitute for walking.

Short 2 to 5 Minute Workouts to Boost Circulation

Many of us have jobs involving long periods of inactivity. After 2 or 3 hours of inactive sitting, rigidity sets in and the brain can become foggy. The remedy for this is a short 2 to 5 minute aerobic workout. I typically walk around for a few minutes, but any repetitive exercise using your arms and legs is acceptable. Another variant is to do jumping jacks and pushups, but the short workout does not need to be that vigorous. If you stop at 2 to 5 minutes, you should prevent breaking out in a sweat, yet still get the blood circulating again.

6. Multipath Rejuvenation Supplements

"The doctor of the future will no longer treat the human frame with drugs, but rather will cure and prevent disease with nutrition."

- Thomas Edison

Summary: Multipath Rejuvenation Supplements

The number and effectiveness of nutritional supplements has increased greatly in the last 20 years. In the not too distant past, the conventional wisdom was that nutritional supplements are unneeded at best and possibly harmful at worst. Indeed, this is still the conventional wisdom among many doctors and experts. However, two recent theories suggest that supplementation can help: **Triage Theory** and the **Evolutionary Theory of Aging**. Triage Theory proposes that sub-optimal levels of many required natural substances lead to preferred substance use by the body for immediate life-critical metabolic needs while starving body processes that require the substance for longer term needs, leading to later chronic heath and aging issues. Evolutionary Aging Theories propose that aging reduces natural selection for genes needed for optimal fitness and health in older animals as reproduction wanes. In other words, natural selection optimizes fitness in the rapidly reproducing young, but mostly ignores fitness in the old that have greatly reduced the production of viable offspring. If either of these two theories is correct, then **Multipath**

Rejuvenation (MuR) dietary supplements that return older adult gene expression to a more youthful state should extend fitness and longevity. Thus, one may use MuR supplements to fine tune gene expression to youthful levels of fitness.

Much new research in the last 20 years has demonstrated that some nutritional supplements are required to reduce substance deficiencies and/or inflammation, while others stimulate your own regenerative stem cells. The favored compounds with the most science behind them are listed below.

1. Vitamin D3 at doses of 2000 to 5000 units per day appears to be one vitamin that can really make a difference in health status. The correct D3 dose for you should be selected based on blood tests showing D3 levels in the ideal range of 40 to 60 ng per ml.
2. Vitamin K2 at a dose of 1 to 6 mg/day acts to promote critical calcium binding proteins.
3. Calcium is known to be a critical mineral in bone formation and many metabolic reactions. Take 600 to 1200 mg/day.
4. Magnesium at 300 to 600 mg per day is required for many metabolic enzymes, muscle activity, and bone growth. Most adults are deficient in this important mineral.
5. Chelated zinc at 15 to 30 mg/day is a critical mineral for bone growth, skin, and immunity.
6. Chelated selenium at 50 to 100 mcg/day and chelated chromium at 200 mcg/day have positive effects on gene regulation and metabolism. Both may be taken with other chelated trace minerals such as: 1 mg

copper, 1 mg manganese, 50 mcg molybdenum, 150 mcg iodine, 2 mg iron, and 2 mg boron.

7. Lithium salts (1 to 5 mg/day) have been linked to longer lifespans.
8. Alpha-lipoic acid at 50 to 100 mg/day reduces inflammation.
9. Co-Q10 at 75 to 150 mg/day reduces inflammation.
10. Omega-3 fish oil with at least 600 mg/day of EPA/DHA reduces inflammation.
11. Astaxanthin at 4 to 8 mg/day reduces skin inflammation.
12. Lutein at 10 to 20 mg/day reduces eye inflammation.
13. Curcumin at 800-1000 mg/day reduces neural inflammation.
14. Kyolic 104 garlic extract at 1-2 capsules per day reduces systemic inflammation.
15. **Supplements that** stimulate your own regenerative stem cells.
16. Multipath Rejuvenation (MuR) dietary supplements to support memory, thinking, coordination, and stimulate stem cells.

Can Supplements Improve Health And Longevity?

Many people and some professionals believe that someone who eats a well-balanced diet of wholesome food does not need to take nutritional supplements. One obvious problem with this viewpoint is that few people in the US eat enough naturally grown whole fruit and vegetables that would provide these essential nutritional factors. Many studies have shown extraordinary gains in health, prevention of disease, and even life extension by treating with supplemental natural substances. Yet many believe that it is unnatural or unnecessary to take nutritional supplements. This is largely contradicted by a growing body of scientific studies. Unfortunately, there are thousands of studies, which often contradict each other, so those who doubt the efficacy of supplements feel justified in their cautious approach. Nevertheless, any thorough study of the literature will uncover compounds that are safe and effective in slowing aging and/or preventing disease.

Before getting into the list of beneficial natural substances, I should mention two novel theories that strongly point to supplementation as a potential way to slow aging and age-related diseases. First, there is the **Evolutionary Theory of Aging** that proposes that aging occurs because natural selection screens for optimal genetic fitness in the fertile young, but that fitness declines as fertility wanes at later ages. In agreement with the theory, it has been determined that **hundreds of genes have altered expression with age**. Most significantly, most, if not all, treatments that slow aging appear to delay or reverse senescent gene expression. The problem is that there are scores of important genes that change expression with age, so no one treatment or life style change will do all that needs to be done to correct the trajectory of progressively more unfit gene expression with age. Therefore, the Evolutionary Theory of Aging suggest **Multipath Rejuvenation (MuR)** supplementation with many synergistic substances targeting critical age-sensitive genes might be a viable strategy to slow, stop, or even reverse aspects of aging.

The second theoretic reason for taking MuR supplements is Bruce Ames' **Triage Theory, which states that scarce supplies of required micro-nutrients are** *prioritized to maximizing short-term survival at the expense of long-term survival (aging).* This type of triage allocation mechanism likely developed via natural selection to deal with shortages of vital nutrients. Thus, natural selection favors genetic mutations in proteins that boost survival in the young and fertile even if that means other proteins that favor long term survival are curtailed.

For example, if not enough calcium is available in the diet, the body releases calcium from bones into the blood circulation to maintain the required metabolic levels of calcium in most cells, but this leads to the long term problem of osteoporosis if the scarcity of calcium becomes chronic. The release of other essential minerals like magnesium and zinc from bone also occurs with scarcity of these minerals and these mineral losses can also lead to osteoporosis.

Other examples of similar metabolic trade-offs that accelerate age associated diseases occur with the many vital proteins using Vitamin K and selenium as cofactors. Those cofactor proteins that are not needed for short term survival are down regulated even though aging and the decline in long term fitness is accelerated. These examples are not the exception, but likely the norm for those natural substances that are required for multiple vital processes and subject to scarcity due to variable diet. *Even in the case where the body synthesizes the required natural substance, the aged or injured body may not produce enough of the self-generated substance leading to localized scarcity that further promotes aging. In this case, daily supplementation with the substance could alleviate the scarcity and minimize or avoid the long range damage.*

Given that MuR supplementation is desirable for slowing aging and promoting health, there is still the question of when supplementation should start. The desirable time to begin MuR supplementation is likely to be around 25 years of age when the long term effects of nutritional scarcity are beginning to be felt. However, MuR supplementation really becomes essential by the age of 40. Of course, for the majority of young people who have poor diets in their teen years, supplementation with minerals and some other nutrients would be beneficial.

MuR Triage Supplements to Reduce Age Deficiencies

Unless you are outside in the sun without sunscreen protection on a daily basis, the most important MuR supplement may be **Vitamin D3**, which has a hormone like action in humans that is essential for many protective functions. It may surprise you to read that many adults over 30 are deficient in Vitamin D and that the long term effects of this deficiency can impair your immune system, and increase your risk of heart disease and cancer. Like our ancestors at all ages, most children sans sunscreen lotion get enough sun exposure in the summer to produce 10,000 units or more of Vitamin D per day. But adults in western societies often drastically limit their sun exposure without sunscreen protection and are mostly indoors during the day. Therefore, many people are significantly deficient in this critical vitamin.

The best way to determine if you are deficient in Vitamin D is with a blood test to check if your blood level is in the desirable range. The ideal level is 50 to 60 ng/ml. If the blood level is below 30 ng/ml, then you are dangerously deficient and likely have increased risks of bone loss, poor immunity, inflammation, and cancer. Supplement with 2000 units of Vitamin D3 per day for 6 months and then retest your Vitamin D level. If still below 40 ng/ml, consult with your doctor. You may increase your Vitamin D3 level to 4000 or 5000 units per day for 6 months or more, which should get you in the desirable range. Vitamin D3 at up to 6000 units/day is generally safe to take long term, but every two years it is best to have your Vitamin D3 blood level tested and consult your doctor if your levels are outside the desired range. Also note that Vitamin D3 soft gels in oil are more bioavailable than are the solid forms in capsules.

Vitamin K2 is another essential MuR vitamin that promotes several vital calcium binding proteins. For example, **Osteocalcin** plays a critical role in placing minerals in bone and **Matrix Gla Proteins (MGPs)** inhibit calcification in most body tissues including blood vessels. With age, calcium often exits the bone to make up for calcium deficiencies in the tissues. If various calcium binding proteins are suppressed in activity due to Vitamin K2 deficiency, the calcium is deposited into soft tissues instead of bone, promoting calcification of organs and blood vessels. Needless to say, tissue calcification is not good and leads to loss of function in organs and hardening of arteries (arteriosclerosis). But much of this damage is minimized if Vitamin D3 and K2 levels are sufficient. Vitamin K comes in both K1 and K2 versions with K2 being the most important. Supplement with 1 to 6 mg/day of Vitamin K2 if you are 40 or older.

Note that Vitamin K2 also comes in two commercial forms (MK4 and MK7), which differ as to the length of the carbon tail. Purists think that MK7 is the best form of Vitamin K2, but MK4 is more economical and found naturally in most animals and in food sources. Moreover, most clinical trials with high doses of Vitamin K2 have used the MK4 version of Vitamin K2 with positive outcomes. I have taken high 5 mg/day doses of the MK4 version of Vitamin K2 for several years and my dentist has noticed improved bone growth around my teeth with gum/tooth pockets in the youthful 2-3 mm range.

Calcium is a key mineral in the body with essential roles in bone, muscle, and neurons. Most people get the bulk of their calcium from dairy products, which are not generally recommended for adults because of high animal protein content. While fruit and vegetables have calcium, the levels are too low to ensure that you get enough calcium. Thus, it is best to supplement with calcium supplements (e.g. Tums) of 600 to 1200 mg/day. If you do take calcium supplements, it is also important to take Vitamin K2 and D3 (see above) to avoid excess calcification of your organs and blood vessels that often occurs with age.

Magnesium is another essential mineral that plays a major role in health. But unlike calcium, magnesium is not enriched in most foods (nuts are a good magnesium source) and many people are deficient in this critical mineral, especially if they live in a soft water area with low mineral content. Magnesium uptake is in competition with calcium uptake, so an imbalance of either mineral can create a deficiency of the other. Magnesium is a MuR cofactor for many body processes and deficiencies can lead to bone loss, muscle weakness, irregular heartbeat, hypertension, insomnia, tiredness, unsteady gait, etc. Most people would benefit from supplementing with 300 to 600 mg/day of magnesium together with 600 to 1200 mg/day of calcium. If you get intestinal problems with magnesium, it is recommended to take magnesium along with calcium and/or take chelated magnesium.

Zinc is an essential trace mineral that accompanies calcium and magnesium in the formation of bone. Zinc is also a MuR cofactor in gene regulation, growth, and insulin activity. An impaired sense of taste and smell, poor immunity, hair loss, low energy, poor memory, infertility, slow wound healing, ringing in the ears, and skin problems are also linked to zinc deficiency Like magnesium, zinc is greatly reduced in modern food processing with white flour having only 23% of the natural level of zinc. Adults should supplement with 15 to 30 mg of chelated zinc per day.

Selenium is another essential trace mineral that is sometimes deficient due to modern food processing methods and/or food grown on selenium deficient soil. Selenium is a MuR cofactor in genetic regulation and metabolism, so it has effects on many molecular pathways. Deficiencies of selenium have been linked to arthritis, cancer, cataracts, dermatitis, dementia, heart disease, inflammation, insomnia, irritability, and wrinkles. Most adults will benefit from supplementing with 50 to 100 mcg of chelated selenium, but it may not be advisable to supplement with higher doses. *Selenium is best taken with chelated zinc and other chelated trace minerals at moderate daily doses: 1 mg copper, 1 mg manganese, 50 mcg molybdenum, 150 mcg iodine, 2 mg iron, and 2 mg boron.*

There is another very important trace mineral that is rarely found in nutritional supplements, but apparently quite important for longevity: 1-5 mg of lithium as **lithium orotate** or **lithium aspartate**. Lithium has been linked to longer lifespan in both animals and humans. Other studies have shown that lithium can actually rejuvenate or amplify neurons in the brain, while providing neuroprotection from environmental toxins. Lithium may also help with Alzheimer's disease, dementia, glaucoma, attention deficit disorder, and depression.

As a final trace mineral, supplement with 200 mcg of **chelated chromium**. Chromium is important in glucose metabolism. As a MuR component, it may provide some protection against Alzheimer's disease and diabetes.

Supplements to Reduce Inflammation

Acute inflammation is the natural response of the immune system to injury or infection and it is important mechanism for healing. However, chronic or low-grade systemic inflammation is not favorable for health and longevity. Indeed, for some experts, *systemic low-grade inflammation has become the "Unified Field Theory" explanation for disease*, because of clear linkage of inflammation to many diverse diseases such as Alzheimer's, autoimmune diseases, arthritis, atherosclerosis, cancer, celiac disease, prostatitis, type II diabetes, and heart disease. Inflammation is also thought to play a role in the frailty and functional decline that often accompanies aging.

A key biomarker for chronic inflammation is a blood protein called *C-Reactive Protein (CRP)*, which is produced in the liver in response to systemic inflammation. High levels of CRP are an indicator of increased risk for high LDL cholesterol and heart disease. You should discuss with your doctor if your CRP level is above 1.

Unfortunately, chronic inflammation appears to be all too common in individuals past 30 or 40 years of age. Chronic inflammation is a complicated process with many causes. The first line of defense is a good diet of mostly whole foods and low animal protein, while minimizing omega-6 oils and trans fats. Additionally, MuR supplements are valuable in controlling chronic inflammation. Below is a list of the best anti-inflammatory supplements with a good track record in reducing inflammation and promoting health.

Alpha-lipoic acid acts to reduce IL-6 levels (another measure of inflammation) and can inhibit the ability of inflammatory white blood cells to divide or adhere to the lining of blood vessels, which is a primary cause of atherosclerosis. Moreover, many studies have shown that alpha-lipoic acid can block the inflammatory effects of many experimental treatments. Note that alpha-lipoic is a natural molecule produced in human cells and active in mitochondria. Yet it is often found at sub-optimal doses in the inefficient mitochondria of older adults, which typically produce oxidative stress byproducts.

Since alpha-lipoic acid is lipid soluble, it accumulates over a period of months with daily intake. Thus, the optimal dose of alpha-lipoic is likely in the 50 to 100 mg/day range, rather than the prevalent commercial 200, 300, or 600 mg/day capsules. These higher doses can reduce effectiveness and increase the risks of unwanted side effects. One such side effect may be suppression of the immune system.

Co-Q10 is another natural substance produced in human cells and active in mitochondria. Low levels of Co-Q10 lead to inefficient mitochondria energy production that generates oxidative stress and subsequent damage to genes, membranes, and mitochondria. In addition, Co-Q10 greatly reduces the pro-inflammatory NF-kB1 gene expression and the release of the inflammatory cytokine TNF-alpha. As Co-Q10 is also lipid soluble, it is best to supplement with Co-Q10 at 75 mg/day to 150 mg/day.

Another essential supplement for lowering inflammation is *omega-3 fish oil*, which reduces inflammatory cytokines such as IL-6 and TNF-alpha. The most beneficial substances in fish oil are the purified essential omega-3 fatty acids eicosapentaenoic acid (EPA) and docasahexaenoic acid (DHA) that raise good HDL cholesterol while lowering LDL cholesterol and triglycerides. Although humans synthesize EPA and DHA from required omega-3 oils, most diets have too little omega-3 oils and the EPA/DHA synthesizing capacity is of variable efficiency in different people. The recommendation is to get at least 600 mg/day of EPA/DHA. Pharmaceutical grade fish oil is the best but is more costly. Also note that omega-6 oils are pro-inflammatory, so you will require more anti-inflammatory omega-3 oils if you consume the inflammatory omega-6 rich diet of the typical American. However, you can also ingest too much omega-3, as overdosing with fish oil can suppress the immune system.

Astaxanthin is a carotenoid that gives the reddish color in krill, crayfish, salmon meat, and flamingo birds. As a purified supplement, astaxanthin is typically purified from algae or is synthesized. Astaxanthin possesses potent MuR antioxidant and anti-inflammatory activity, which is partly due to its capacity to suppress pro-inflammatory genes. Clinical trials have shown a marked ability to prevent sunburn from ultraviolet sunlight with a dose of only 4 mg/day. Based on its proven ability to block skin damage from ultraviolet rays, astaxanthin has a strong anti-inflammatory benefit for skin, and may also be anti-inflammatory internally as well. I recommend 4 to 8 mg/day of astaxanthin from the natural algae source.

Lutein is another anti-inflammatory carotenoid that is found in many vegetables and fruit. Lutein, and to a lesser extent the isomeric carotenoid *zeaxanthin*, are the two major carotenoid pigments found in the retina. Both lutein and zeaxanthin are thought to function by blocking light damage to the cornea and eye tissue. Clinical trials have shown lutein and zeaxanthin to be effective in preventing various eye diseases, including macular degeneration, cataracts, and retinitis pigmentosa. As is the case with astaxanthin, there may be systemic anti-inflammatory effects throughout the body. The recommendation is to take 10 to 20 mg/day of lutein.

Curcumin is a brightly yellow anti-inflammatory substance that comes from the popular spice turmeric root, which is the main flavor in curries from India. *Turmeric root* has been a central player in the Ayurvedic medicine of India for thousands of years and recent research has identified curcumin as the substance with most of the biological activity in turmeric. In both animals and human studies, curcumin has shown anti-amyloid, anti-arthritic, anti-cancer, anti-ischemic, anti-microbial, and anti-inflammatory effects. In India, where curcumin is widely used as a spice, the rate of Alzheimer's disease is strikingly low. Many of curcumin effects may be due to its proven ability to reduce NF-kB, which is a major factor promoting inflammation. Moreover, curcumin has been shown to reduce the size of plaques in the mouse model of Alzheimer's disease.

Despite the many positive effects on diseases in animals and a long history of successful culinary and medicinal use in India, curcumin has not done as well in Western clinical trials. One reason for this is the very poor bioavailability of curcumin in purified extracts. Curcumin rapidly undergoes glucuronidation in humans, which limits its systemic uptake and blocks crossing of the blood-brain barrier. One way around the low bioavailability of curcumin is to include small amounts of *piperine*, which is a pepper extract that inhibits glucuronidation. I recommend 800 to 1000 mg/day of an 85% curcumin extract containing small doses of piperine. While curcumin does not cause significant side effects, some people can experience stomach upset or dizziness at higher doses. Curcumin also reduces blood clotting, so consult your physician if you are taking blood thinners.

Garlic, a vegetable in the onion family, has been used in cooking and medicine in most cultures for thousands of years. Garlic has been used medicinally to treat many disorders, such as hypertension, heart disease, enlarged prostate, arthritis, bacterial and viral infections, and prevention of various cancers. While garlic is well known for its health benefits, the strong odor of garlic breath and occasional stomach upset has reduced the use of whole garlic. The answer to this dilemma was to create a garlic supplement that had the health benefits of whole garlic without the smell and bulk. *Kyolic* is a famous Japanese proprietary *Aged Garlic Extract (AGE)* produced by Wakunaga that has been tested in hundreds of studies, showing that AGE garlic can provide as good or better health benefits than fresh garlic without the odors and side effects. I recommend 2 capsules per day of *Kyolic 104* to help reduce inflammation and boost immunity. Like curcumin, garlic has anticoagulant properties, so consult your physician if you are taking blood thinners.

Supplements to Promote Your Own Stem Cells

In youth, we have a robust ability to repair and regenerate many damaged tissues. As we age, our stem cell populations become depleted and/or slowly lose their capacity to repair. Moreover, the micro-environment around stem cells becomes less nurturing with age, so cell turnover and repair are further reduced. This natural reduction in our healing capacity occurs so slowly that we are barely aware of it, but we start to notice the body changes by our 40s and especially after 50 years of age. Promoting and maintaining our own adult stem cells are critically important for preventing disease, repairing damage, and slowing aging.

To promote our adult stem cells, we need a two pronged approach: 1) slowing the intrinsic aging of our adult stem cell populations, and 2) improving the micro-environment around our stem cells. The first approach is mainly directed at reducing stem cell aging. This involves stabilizing telomere loss and gene expression in stem cells. While **TA-65** was the initial commercial product to help with telomere loss (see http://www.revgenetics.com/ta-65/), there is now an herbal product that provides telomere support: **Stem Cell 100® (SC100)** from Life Code (see http://www.lifecoderx.com/stem-cell-100/). SC100 is a MuR supplement that helps adults regain their youthful regenerative potential by stabilizing telomeres in stem cells. SC100 also promotes adult stem cells by stimulating one of the 4 genes known to potentiate stem cell function. In longevity experiments in model animals, SC100 was able to double maximum lifespan.

The second approach to promoting stem cells is mainly directed at minimizing inflammation and other systemic factors that degrade stem cell micro-environments. The MuR supplement SC100 acts to lower inflammation directly via other pathways. Of course, a good diet and moderate exercise also help lower inflammation and promote telomerase activity at the same time.

While the benefit of SC100 to stem cells would not be immediately apparent, many users have reported beneficial effects including:
1. More endurance during vigorous workouts
2. Higher resistance to colds and flu
3. Lower blood sugar for those in the normal range

4. Lower blood pressure for those in the normal range
5. Lower levels of inflammation
6. Less pain and faster recovery times
7. Loss of belly fat that was resistant to other efforts
8. Younger looking, smoother and more elastic skin
9. Sinus clearing and less chest inflammation
10. Improvements in gum health
11. General mood elevation
12. Improvements in vision

We do not make medical claims for SC100. However, you might find it interesting to do before and after blood tests with your doctor and monitor LDL and HDL cholesterol, fasting glucose, fasting insulin and C-Reactive Protein (CRP) which is an indicator of chronic inflammation. Another test is to periodically check your blood pressure. In field testing, we found that people taking SC100 tended to have significantly higher HDL cholesterol and lower fasting glucose and blood pressure. Note that SC100 is not meant as a treatment or preventive for hypertension, cholesterol problems, diabetes, or inflammation. But SC100 can help with keeping these parameters at more healthful levels for those already in the normal range.

If you are 125 pounds or less or in your 20s, then it is best to only take one capsule of SC100 per day preferably after lunch. For those over 125 pounds and over 30 years of age, we recommend two capsules per day preferably taken at breakfast and dinner.

MuR Supplements to Slow Brain Aging

The central organ that we all want to preserve with age is our brain and associated sensory and neural systems. With many baby boomers reaching their 60s, dementia in all its variant forms is becoming more prevalent. But even if one does not suffer from a chronic dementia disease, "senior moments", clouded thinking, and/or failing eyesight and hearing afflict most people over 60. Can nutritional and herbal supplements help preserve memory, clear thinking, coordination, vision, and hearing as we age?

The surprising answer appears to be that nutritional supplements can help. Recall that aging is caused by many genetic pathways that have not been optimized for fitness with advancing age. The theory is that treating with MuR compounds that act on multiple fitness pathways can reconfigure gene expression in cells to the more optimal state found in youth.

One example of this in the existing scientific literature is **Vitamin K2**, which was mentioned earlier. Besides its role in blood clotting, bone production, and prevention of organ and blood vessel calcification, Vitamin K2 proteins also have important roles in the central nervous system (CNS). For example, the **Gas6 gene** is a CNS gene that enhances cell survival, cell growth, and myelination. Loss of myelination on neuronal axons is a common occurrence in dementia and normal CNS aging. Another CNS gene requiring Vitamin K2 is **Protein S**, which has potent neuroprotective effects. Vitamin K2 is also essential for **sphingolipids**, which have a major role in the myelin sheath and neuronal membranes. I recommend taking 1 to 6 mg a day of Vitamin K2, which are very high doses.

In our effort at Genescient to identify genes linked to brain aging and dementia, we have identified the critical longevity pathways in long lived *Drosophila* and humans using genomic and machine learning technologies. We then identified drugs and nutritional compounds that act on these critical longevity and neural pathways. Finally, we screened both single compounds and combinations of active compounds that synergistically support longevity and neuronal functions in *Drosophila* models of Alzheimer's disease.

For our screening assay, we used transgenic *Drosophila* that had mutant human genes responsible for early onset Alzheimer's disease. We screened for compounds and combinations of compounds that could suppress dementia that developed with age in these test animals. As a control, we found that an existing human Alzheimer drug (**Mementin**) was active in our *Drosophila* tests, showing that our *Drosophila* assay was a good model for testing human treatments.

The results of our extensive experiments using this screening system was that **we identified a group of eight nutritional components that were able to synergistically suppress the dementia effects of the mutant human beta amyloid and tau genes in this animal model.** We have filed a patent on this formulation and this group of eight components is now undergoing a randomly controlled double blind clinical trial on a small group of moderate to severe Alzheimer's patients.

Because the eight components are all GRAS substances, the formulation (**Memex 100™**) is now available for sale as a dietary supplement for memory and neural support. For more information, visit the website http://www.LifeCodeRx.com/memex100/.

Following Your Progression to Health and Longevity

Whenever you are changing your diet, exercise, or supplement regimes, it is advisable to measure your progress toward better health and longevity. To measure progress accurately, it is necessary to have biomarker metrics that follow your progression. Below I list several simple tests that can be used.

The first biomarkers are **blood pressure** and **pulse rate**, which are general metrics of your mortality risks. For this purpose, I recommend purchasing an automatic blood pressure monitor such as the Omron HEM-711ACN2. It is best to take your blood pressure and pulse early in the morning when you first wake up, as blood pressure tends to be highest at that time. Readings of 115 over 75 mm of Hg or lower are desirable. Pulse rate should be 60 beats per minute or less for men and 66 or less for women.

Another simple marker that you can do yourself is **reaction speed**, which normally tracks with cognition and thinking speed. As you might expect, genetic factors do affect an individual's reaction speed. However, your reaction speed typically peaks in the late teens and often declines very slowly thereafter. Diet, exercise, and MuR supplements can also affect reaction speed, so it is best to monitor your reaction speed periodically to determine if it is improving, staying the same, or declining. A simple online computer test for reaction speed can be found on the website http://www.bbc.co.uk/science/humanbody/sleep/sheep/reaction_version5.swf Get your best average of 5 tries and keep a record to follow your progress taking supplements and/or in the changes to your lifestyle.

Skin cell turnover declines with age. Therefore, in a baby, skin cells die and are replaced every 2 weeks and in teenagers skin cell replacement occurs in about 3 to 4 weeks. By the time we reach 50, cell turnover has typically slowed to 2 to 3 months. That is why skin healing is so slow when we are older and why skin gets thin and loses elasticity with age. You can monitor skin aging and how your life style and supplements are affecting your rate of skin aging by performing several of the skin tests described below.

For example, the *"Skin Pinch Test"* is a simple characteristic to monitor skin aging. If one pinches the skin on the back of the hand and then releases it, older skin takes much longer to return to its previous state. ***Pinch the skin on the back of your relaxed hand for about 5 seconds, let go, and then time how long the skin takes to return to its previous state.*** In the elastic skin of a child, the pinched out skin returns to its previous smooth state immediately. In someone in their 20s, it can take 1 to 3 seconds, whereas in someone over 50 it may take more than 8 to 10 seconds for the pinched skin to return to its previous state.

Another skin elasticity test is to hold your thigh with both hands and slide your hands closer together to induce skin wrinkling. Be sure to squeeze your skin together to induce wrinkles lengthwise on your thigh and then induce wrinkles across your thigh. The older your skin is (i.e. the slower the skin cell turnover), the more these skin movements generate skin wrinkles. With the right lifestyle and supplements, skin aging can be slowed and even stopped.

One last way to monitor skin cell aging is to check on the number and size of aging skin warts and spots, which can be irregular raised spots or dark colored spots. Aging spots naturally occur with greater frequency as we age. Your local dermatologist can freeze or cut off the unsightly warts and laser bleach skin spots, but you will be fighting an unwinnable war without good nutrition and MuR supplements to regenerate skin stem cells from the inside.

Other aging markers are determined by laboratory blood testing. A key lab biomarker is blood glucose. Blood glucose should be in the range of 70 to 100, but between 75 and 90 is most desirable. A second lab biomarker is C-Reactive Protein (CRP), which should be much less than 1. A third lab biomarker is Vitamin D3 level which should be in the range of 40 to 80 ng/ml with the ideal range of 40 to 60 ng/ml. Finally, HDL and LDL cholesterol should be tested. Ideally, HDL should be above 60 and LDL should be below 80, but those cholesterol levels are difficult to attain without a very good diet and/or statin drugs.

7. Model Systems for Studying Aging

"In both mice and men, during adult life span, aging causes an exponential increase in vulnerability to almost all pathologies."

- David Harrison

Aging is defined as a gradual change in an organism that leads to increased risk of frailty, disease, and death. Model systems have provided important tools for uncovering the drivers of the aging process.

Model Systems for Studying Aging	*S. Cerevisciae* (yeast)	*C. Elegans* (worm)
	D. Melanogaster (fly)	Mutant mice
	Primates (monkey)	Human cell senescence
	Progeroid humans	Centenarians

Our current understanding of aging has come from the use of different model systems of aging: yeast, worms, flies, rodents (e.g. mice), non-human primates, human progeroid syndromes, human centenarians, and human cells in culture. One major advantage of using differing systems is that all of the modern techniques of genetics and molecular biology can be fully employed. In addition, there is a marked advantage of using those systems amenable to experimentation so that various theories of aging can be rigorously tested and falsified. Moreover, genetic expression and functional changes can be easily followed in many of these aging models, so as to pinpoint the critical genetic and functional components of the aging process.

Before launching into a discussion of the current model systems for studying aging, **we need to define precisely what aging is**. One complicating factor in defining aging is that many changes once thought to be intrinsic to aging are now recognized as effects of underlying degenerative disease. Uncoupling the age-related diseases from general aging process is no simple undertaking. Alzheimer's disease is a good example of this problem. Beta-amyloid plaques and tau tangles are characteristic of Alzheimer's disease, but are also typically observed in the healthy elderly that have few of the Alzheimer's symptoms. Are plaques and tangles indicators of normal aging or a disease process? No one has a definitive answer to that question. While it is certainly true that the risk of Alzheimer's disease climbs rapidly for those individuals over 70, the role that the aging process itself plays in Alzheimer's disease is still an open area of research.

Given the above caveats, a good definition of aging is given by the Britannica Concise Encyclopedia: **Aging is a "gradual change in an organism that leads to increased risk of weakness, disease, and death".** Note that this definition is similar to the observation by David Harrison that aging in both mice and men causes an exponential increase in vulnerability to almost all pathologies. The actual declines in function with age occur at the cell, organ, and systemic levels, which is not to say that all cells, organs, and systems are affected equally. Genetic and environmental influences can differentially impact certain cells, organs, and systems.

This view of aging naturally leads to multiple causes of aging and multipath treatments for delaying aging. We will discuss this in greater detail in later chapters, but in this chapter we will explore the model systems that have yielded data on the aging process and life span extension in various species.

Budding yeast (*Saccharomyces cerevisciae*) are the simplest organism used in aging studies. Budding yeast are most commonly used to make beer or bread, but have long been used in genetic research. While yeast lack the complexity of multicellular organisms, each young budding yeast cell can only undergo a limited number of cell divisions (their replicative lifespan) before the progeny become progressively enlarged and finally stop dividing. The replicative lifespan of yeast is determined by many environmental and genetic factors, as is the case for higher organisms. For example, *calorie restriction* (reduced calorie diet) is an environmental change that extends replicative lifespan in yeast cells. Calorie restriction has been observed to extend lifespan in every species for which it has been tested, including yeast cells, making these one-celled animals an appropriate model for clues to understanding aging.

Nematode worms (*Caenorhabditis elegans*) are simple multicellular animals (only 959 cells per worm) with a normal lifespan of 11 to 20 days depending on incubation temperature. Because of the ease of making genetic mutants and its short lifespan, *C. elegans* was one of the first organisms to be used in genetic studies of aging. Dozens of longevity genes that dramatically increase worm lifespan have been identified using this organism. The down side to the study of worm aging is that *C. elegans* is a simple invertebrate animal and, like yeast, is a species that is far removed from humans. Nevertheless, nematodes respond to calorie restriction with extended lifespan as do other animals and many of the identified longevity assurance genes are likely active participants in human aging.

Fruit flies (*Drosophila melanogaster*) are far more complex that nematodes or yeast. *Drosophila* also has some 100,000 neurons, which makes the fly brain much closer to mammals than nematodes that only have a few hundred neurons. Some transgenic Drosophila (with inserted human neural disease genes) have provided good models for Alzheimer's disease and Parkinson's disease.

While *Drosophila* fruit flies are much smaller than the common house fly, *Drosophila* has been extensively studied for years in both developmental biology and aging research since they are easy to alter genetically and have a relatively short life span. As is the case with yeast and worms, flies are evolutionally distant from both mammals and humans. Yet, flies have extended lifespan on dietary restriction and age-related genes have been identified in flies that are conserved in yeast, worms, mice and humans. *Drosophila* has been studied extensively by evolutionary biologists, who have developed very long lived lines of **Methuselah flies** that live 3 to 4 times longer than wild flies. We have also used *Drosophila* as a powerful model system to study the effects of supplements and drugs on longevity (111), which in later unpublished work has led to novel multi-component MuR supplements for longevity.

The **mouse** and other rodents have long been used in aging studies. Currently, the mouse is the preferred rodent for aging studies because of their small size and the ease of producing genetic knockouts. Of course, mice are mammals, which make them much closer in evolution to humans than are yeasts, worms, or flies. Indeed, mice are currently used as the preferred animal models for investigating many human diseases. In the aging field, many genetic mutant mice have been used to test for lifespan extension of selected genes. The National Institutes of Health (NIH) has contracted for three academic labs (University of Texas at San Antonio, University of Michigan, and Jackson Labs) to use various mice strains to test drugs and compounds that are candidates for lifespan extension.

The comparison of aging in mice with aging in yeast, nematodes, and flies has provided valuable information on the mechanisms of aging that appear common to all animals (so called 'public' aging, as opposed to 'private' or species-specific aging). A summary of these exciting experiments will be given in the next chapter.

Primates are the closest class of species to humans. Unfortunately, primates are large animals with long lifespans (8 to 40 years). This makes aging research on primates expensive and results are very slow in coming. The major use of primates in aging research has been the testing of calorie restriction. The first experiment in testing Rhesus monkeys for the effects of calorie restriction started in the 1990s, but has not gone on long enough to obtain complete lifespan data. However, the data obtained so far indicates a slowing of aging by calorie restriction in Rhesus monkeys.

Human progeroid syndromes are a heterogeneous class of disorders with clinical features that mimic accelerated aging in humans. Werner syndrome and Hutchinson-Gilford progeria are the most studied progeroid syndromes as potential models of accelerated aging. In the case of Werner syndrome, individuals with the disease appear to age very rapidly in their 40s, whereas individuals with Hutchinson-Gilford progeria start aging rapidly as young children and typically die in their teens of one or more of the age-related diseases. Several gene mutations largely responsible for these two progeroid syndromes are now known and may provide valuable insight into the aging process.

On the opposite side of human aging spectrum are the long lived **Centenarians**, who survive to be 100 years and older and **Super Centenarians**, who survive to 110 and older. Centenarians and Super Centenarians fall into two classes: escapers and survivors. Escapers typically have genetic advantages that help them avoid any serious age related disease, whereas survivors have suffered through one or more age-related disease. Genetic studies of the centenarian populations as compared to normal young and old humans are beginning to bear some fruit, but obtaining appropriate controls has posed challenges.

The final model for studying aging is the proliferative (dividing) capacity of **human cells in culture.** It has been known for some 50 years that human fibroblasts have a limited division capacity of about 50 to 70 doublings in culture. As this replicative capacity is reached, the cells get progressively enlarged (like old yeast cells) and finally lose their capacity to divide in a process called **cell aging** or **cell senescence**. These late replicative cells also do not function as well as cells with few doublings. Using this model we have shown that cells aging in culture change their gene expression pattern to a more senescent state (110), indicating that the **body appears to age at the cellular level**.

Although many have doubted the role of cell aging, it is worth noting that cells from Werner syndrome and Hutchinson-Gilford progeria patients have less potential for replicative division than cells from normal patients, which correlates with their shorter lifespans. Other work to be described later shows that cell aging is related to the problem of telomere loss.

The above brief description of the major lines of research in aging begs the question of the relevance of the different models to human aging. Although each of the above model systems has its critics, the consensus view of the experts is that all of the models mentioned above have some relevance to human aging and, taken together, give us the most comprehensive understanding of the aging process that is available with today's technologies.

8. The Genetics of Lifespan

"Longevity has a strong genetic component, as has become apparent from studies with a variety of organisms, from yeast to humans."

- **J. Vijg and Y. Suh**

Summary: The Genetics of Lifespan

There are at least eight dissimilar genetic pathways involved in longevity: 1) Insulin/ IGF1 signaling; 2) Mitochondrial stability; 3) Oxidative stress defense; 4) Genomic stability; 5) Extracellular Matrix; 6) Cell growth/Autophagy; 7) Inflammation; and 8) Ion/Lipid transport. The genetic data on longevity that is summarized in this chapter generate a very important principle: ***Any intervention to slow aging should act via Multipath Rejuvenation (MuR) treatments to have an optimal impact on slowing the aging process.***

The lifespan of worms (*C. elegans*) has been extended 100% or more by modifications of a single gene (19, 38). For example, reduction in the expression of genes age-1 or daf-2 typically doubles worm lifespan. These two genes are cell membrane receptors in the insulin-like hormone signaling pathway that regulates the response to starvation (17). Other genes in this insulin-like signaling pathway such as the FOXO Forkhead transcription factors and Sir-2 (a histone deacetylase) also regulate lifespan (13, 57). It is difficult to overemphasize the role of insulin-like genes in aging, because the insulin-like pathway acts on multiple genes and is highly conserved throughout evolution in yeast, worms, flies, and rodents (25, 27, 32-33). The insulin-like genes also include insulin-signaling itself, as deletion of one of the two copies of the insulin receptor substrate 2 (IRS-2) in mice leads to extended mouse lifespan (5).

It is important to note that all of the data on insulin-like genes indicate that extended lifespan comes from *reducing* the natural activity of the insulin-like pathway. In applying this to humans, an apparent contradiction arises from the fact that humans with insufficient insulin levels or impaired insulin sensitivity suffer from diabetes and typically have an earlier appearance of many of the age related diseases and shortened lifespan. Understanding this inconsistency may illuminate how the insulin-like pathway extends lifespan.

The apparent contradiction may be understood by comparing the two types of diabetics: Early-onset type I diabetes and late-onset type II diabetes. In type I diabetics, the pancreas has lost most or all of its ability to make insulin and therefore type I diabetics require periodic insulin injections to live. Unfortunately, with periodic injections it is not possible to regulate the insulin level as is naturally done by the pancreas, which continuously adjusts the amount of secreted insulin to maintain a constant level of blood glucose. Blood insulin levels surge right after injection and slowly fall until the next injection. Under these conditions, the patient's insulin levels will sometimes be abnormally high and other times abnormally low. In rodents it has been shown that reducing insulin levels by half or more is beneficial, but that insulin is an essential hormone, so a certain threshold level of insulin is required (32). Therefore, it is likely that both abnormally low and abnormally high levels of insulin increase the risks of disease and death in type I diabetics.

About 90% of all diabetics have late-onset type II diabetes, which usually appears in those over 50 years of age. The disease develops as a result of the inability of many cells in the body to take up glucose normally, so the levels of blood glucose rise. The pancreas responds to this high blood glucose situation by increasing the level of insulin. As the disease progresses, the cells become increasingly insulin resistant to ever higher levels of insulin, which leads to constitutive high glucose and high insulin levels. It is these conditions of high constitutive insulin levels that apparently lead to age-related diseases (e. g. cardiovascular, Alzheimer's, and some cancers) and shortened life. In the final stages of type II diabetes, the pancreas becomes exhausted by progressively higher insulin requirements, and insulin levels plummet, leading to a condition resembling type I diabetes with the subsequent need for insulin injections.

Besides insulin, **growth hormone (GH)** and the **insulin-like growth factor 1 (IGF1)** are also highly conserved players in the insulin-like pathway (aka the **insulin/IGF1 pathway**) and important factors in longevity. Partial disruption of the GH/IGF1 axis can increase lifespan and insulin sensitivity in worms, flies, and mice (67). For example, **studies have shown that mice missing either the GH gene or GH receptor live substantially longer and have slower cognitive decline** (6, 14, 24, 39). This GH/IGF1 axis is apparently conserved in humans, as women with poorer GH/IGF1 scores have lower body height and improved survival in old age (71). Taking all the data into account, **the insulin/IGF1 pathway clearly plays a major role in the** *aging process and provides major targets for slowing aging and reducing the risks of many age-related diseases*.

Many other gene pathways have been suggested as key factors in aging. The antioxidant enzymes *catalase, glutathione peroxidase (GPx), superoxide dismutase (SOD)* are examples of genes that counteract oxidative stress. Oxidative stress has long been believed by many researchers to be a causative factor in aging, but the specific role of individual endogenous antioxidant enzymes in aging has been controversial. For example, modest over-expression of catalase in flies has no apparent effect on lifespan (53), but massive over-expression of catalase in mitochondria of mouse trangenics increases lifespan significantly (45). *Transgenic flies* (genetically modified flies) over-expressing copper/zinc SOD also have longer lifespans (1), but 50% under-expression of GPx-4 in *transgenic mice* (genetically modified mice) leads to longer lifespan (58). Comparing antioxidant enzymes in short and long lived rodents (3), it appears that the endogenous antioxidants typically play a limited role in the aging process, which is consistent with the mixed results of transgenic experiments (inserting foreign genes for antioxidant enzymes).

While these results suggest that oxidative stress plays only a minor role in longevity, worm lifespan is negatively correlated with oxygen tension (34), which implies a role for oxidative stress in aging since hyper-oxygen environments greatly increase oxidative stress. Oxidative stress is also a well known cause of age-related disease (2).

About 90% of oxygen radicals are generated inside the cell by mitochondria. *Significantly, mitochondrial function declines with age and oxygen radicals increase with age* (28, 36). Rates of oxygen radical leakage from mitochondria are negatively correlated with lifespan in six mammalian species (69). Moreover, systematic genetic screens for longevity in worms have identified genes involved in regulating mitochondria as major modulators of lifespan (15, 29, 43). These data and other results indicate that mitochondrial function and subsequent leaked oxygen radicals are both associated with aging (43). Therefore, it appears that *the role of oxidative stress in aging is associated with mitochondrial function.*

While the insulin/IGF1 and oxidative/mitochondrial pathways have particularly strong effects on the lifespans of nearly all animal species, the genetic data demonstrate that other genes and pathways play a role in the lifespans of selected species. One gene pathway that appears to be important for many species is the pathway for maintaining DNA telomere repeats at the ends of chromosomes. Telomere repeats are critical for maintaining chromosome stability and are slowly lost via cell division or DNA damage due to oxygen radicals. The principle enzyme involved in maintaining telomere repeats (e.g. TTAGGG is the human telomere repeat) is *telomerase*, which has both RNA and protein components.

In the mid-1990s I was a senior scientist working with Geron Corporation when we discovered the RNA component of human and mouse telomerase, as reported in *Science* (9, 21, 31). The discovery was heralded nationally in many major newspapers because of the potential of telomerase drugs as therapeutics for various cancers (77). Anti-cancer telomerase therapeutics are presently in clinical trials.

Telomerase also offers the potential for therapeutics for age-related diseases (26). For example, deficiencies in telomerase correlate with hypertension and higher risks for cardiovascular disease (20, 56). Humans with telomere dysfunctions (e.g. Dyskeratosis congenita) and transgenic mice lacking telomerase have a decreased lifespan and a premature loss of cell renewal (8, 30, 46). The loss of cell renewal is likely the result of the inability of telomerase-deficient stem cells to regenerate tissues (8, 46) and could play a role in many age-related disabilities and diseases.

Telomere maintenance is actually part of a general pathway for **genomic stability, *wherein the genome is protected against genetic damage by oxidation, irradiation, deletions, insertions, and copying errors*.** As it turns out, other members of the genomic stability pathway are also important for longevity. The genome consists of the total set of genes (nuclear DNA and DNA-packaging proteins) that provide a blueprint for every cell in an organism. ***DNA damage accumulates with age*** (47, 66) and this has long been proposed as a significant cause of aging. The recent findings from the human progeria syndromes provide suggestive evidence for the role of DNA damage in aging. For example, Werner's syndrome patients have a defective DNA repair helicase (used to untwist DNA during copying) and thus accumulate DNA damage faster with age than normal humans (65). This enhanced DNA damage leads to conditions of rapid decline of the patient starting in their 40s that mimics premature aging.

Hutchinson-Gilford progeria syndrome is a more general example of genomic instability and aging. Patients with this rare form of progeria appear to age rapidly starting in early childhood and typically suffer premature death as teenagers. The vast majority of patients with Hutchinson-Gilford progeria syndrome produce defective ***lamin A (progerin)*** that improperly binds chromosomes in the nucleus to cause genome instability (49). With the Hutchinson-Gilford progeria, the defective lamin A inhibits cell cycle progression and promotes premature cell aging. Though Hutchinson-Gilford progeria and Werner's syndrome are both rare genetic diseases, their age-like symptoms support the role of genomic stability in aging. Significantly, defective lamin A is present in normal people and defective Lamin A is more prevalent with age.

One more important link to genomic stability that should be noted: Although mitochondria have their own mitochondrial DNA, the vast majority of mitochondrial proteins are coded by nuclear genes. As the nuclear genomic damage accumulates with age, the nuclear genes for mitochondrial proteins risk becoming progressively more mutated. This may be a significant cause of mitochondria decline with age. Moreover, as mitochondria decline in function, they also leak more oxidative radicals that further damage the genomic DNA and mitochondria. This feedback between DNA and mitochondrial damage can lead to a vicious cycle whereby dysfunctional mitochondria accumulate and generate more oxidative stress leading to more genomic damage and still more dysfunctional mitochondrial, eventually ending in cell aging. Oxidative free radicals produced by mitochondrial are also linked to enhanced telomere breakage and loss, which increases genomic instability and cell aging by an alternative pathway (63, 75-76).

While the above discussion is focused on genomic DNA, mitochondria have their own DNA, which encodes some mitochondrial genes involved in respiration. The role of mitochondrial DNA damage in cell aging is controversial. However, it is known that the health consequences of inherited mitochondrial DNA mutations include age-related disorders such as muscle weakness, diabetes, kidney failure, heart disease, dementia, and vision problems (18, 41). We will return to the mitochondria-nuclear interactions in a later chapter to explore a potential critical aspect of aging.

Any review of the genomic stability pathway would be remiss without mentioning the role of the DNA damage-sensing genes p53 and p16. In particular, the accumulation of p16 (INK4a) is a robust marker of cellular aging and in vivo skin aging (62) and also contributes to cellular aging (10-11). Both p16 and p53 are known as tumor suppressor genes, because of their strong role in preventing uncontrolled cancer growth. Therefore, the life extension potential of p16 and p53 likely resides in their ability to prevent metastatic cancer.

Centenarians provide another research opportunity to identify age-related genes. With the average human life expectancy at less than 80 years in most countries, living for 100 years or longer is rare. The most consistent gene that has been identified in various centenarian generations is the lipid transport factor apolipoprotein E (ApoE) epsilon 4 (51, 54). In comparison to middle aged humans, centenarians are less likely to have a copy of the ApoE epsilon 4 gene, but instead have the more benign ApoE epsilon 2 allele. Moreover, humans with two copies of the ApoE epsilon 4 allele have higher risks for early onset cardiovascular disease and dementia.

Recently, it has been reported that a Jewish centenarian cohort had an overrepresentation of mutated IGF1 receptor mutations (70). As expected, centenarians with IGF1 receptor mutation also had shortened stature. Recall that partial loss-of-function mutations of the insulin/IGF1 pathway result in lifespan extension in yeast, worms, flies, and mice. The discovery of common IGF1 receptor mutations in some centenarians indicates that loss-of-function IGF1 mutations lead to life extension in humans as well. FOXO3 is another gene in the insulin/IGF1 signaling pathway that has been strongly associated with longevity in

French, German, Italian, Japanese, and Chinese centenarians (4, 23, 44, 55, 79). ***Thus, the insulin-like growth factor pathway appears to regulate lifespan across species with diverse lengths of lifespans from as short as 2 weeks to as long as 120 years.***

The sequencing of the human genome at the beginning of the 21st Century and the technical ability with gene microarrays to look simultaneously at the expression of many genes in tissues from both young and old individuals has permitted the discovery of human gene pathways that are regulated with age in brain, kidney, and muscle (78). Looking at the common pathways shared by brain, kidney, and muscle tissues, there are six genetic pathways that show consistent directional changes in expression with age (see Table on next page). Genes associated with the **extracellular matrix** (152 genes), **cell growth** (29 genes), **compliment activation** (22 genes), and **cytosolic ribosomes** (8 genes) are up-regulated in brain, kidney, and muscle with age.

Genetic Pathway	Age	Genes	Examples
Extracellular Matrix	↑	152	CSPG2, TIMP1
Cell Growth	↑	29	TGFB1, FGFR1
Compliment Activation	↑	22	C1R, DAF
Cytosolic Ribosomal	↑	8	RPL12, RPS19
Chloride Transport	↓	35	CLCN5, GABRA2
Electron Transport*	↓	95	COX7B, UQCRFS1

Gene expression changes with age in humans for brain, kidney, and muscle. For the six genetic pathways shown, expression goes up (↑) or down (↓) with age. *The electron transport genes also have lowered expression in old mice and flies. Examples of expression changes: CSPG2 = chondroitin sulfate proteoglycan 2; TIMP1 = tissue inhibitor of metalloproteinase 1; TGFB1 = transforming growth factor, β 1; FGFR1 = fibroblast growth factor receptor 1; C1R = complement component 1r; DAF = decay accelerating factor; RPL12 = ribosomal protein L12; RPS19 = ribosomal protein S19; CLCN5 = chloride channel 5; GABRA2 = gamma-aminobutyric acid A receptor; COX7B = cytochrome c oxidase subunit VIIb; UQCRFS1 = ubiquinol-cytochrome c reductase, Rieske iron-sulfur polypeptide 1. (Ref. 78)

Unlike most of the genetic mutation experiments presented earlier, gene expression experiments are merely correlations and do not directly answer whether the gene expression changes are causes or effects of aging. For example, mutations that down-regulate the electron transport chain *extend* lifespan in yeast, worms, flies, and mice, so the down-regulation of the electron transport pathway with age may actually be a helpful compensation in old animals that extends lifespan. Likewise, the up-regulation of cytosolic ribosomal gene pathway may be compensating for the decline of protein synthesis and protein turnover with age (64, 68). On the other hand, reductions with age of the chloride transport pathway is likely detrimental, as blood pressure tends to rise with the buildup of chloride ions. Likewise, three of the up-regulated pathways (extracellular matrix, cell growth, and compliment activation) can cause nonionic changes in the *extracellular environment* in older animals that promotes chronic disease and shortens lifespan.

Also prominent in the changed extracellular environment is the *widespread fibrosis* in various organs in which fibrous connective tissue overgrows and impairs tissue function. Along with fibrosis is the decline in *autophagy*, a catabolic process defined as the degradation of cellular components and infectious agents by the lysosomal system. *Increasing autophagy dysfunction and overactive extracellular matrix formation leads to the accumulation of inter- and extra-cellular debris that is not cleared by the system.* The accumulating debris, over-expression of the extracellular matrix material, and excessive compliment activation disturb the *micro-environment around cells*, which typically weakens cellular and tissue function. The disturbed micro-environment also promotes *chronic inflammation*, which further reduces tissue function.

Note that the genes reported in this chapter are not an exhaustive list of all the genes linked to aging in the plethora of genetic reports. Indeed, there are a bewildering number of genes and gene products that have been genetically linked to aging using the various models of aging. Looking at the many papers showing effects of various genes on the aging process, it is often difficult to visualize a clear pattern of the genetic influence on aging. However, when the genes are organized into large genetic pathways, the picture becomes much clearer. *The most important genes for aging can largely be put into eight broad genetic pathways, as seen in the table below.*

Known Genetic Pathways
that affect longevity

Genetic Pathway	Examples
Insulin/IGF1	Insulin, IGF1, receptors
Mitochondrial Stability	COX7B, UQCRFS1
Oxidative Stress Defense	SOD, Catalase, klotho
Genomic Stability	Telomerase, p16, lamin A
Extracellular Matrix	CSPG2, TIMP1
Cell Growth/Autophagy	TGFB1, FGFR1, HSP70
Inflammation	C1R, DAF, IL-6, CRP
Ion/Lipid Transport	CLCN5, GABRA2, APOE, HDL

The genetic pathways important for aging have mostly been explained in the above table, but the last three pathways have been broadened to include related genes. Thus, cell growth is combined with autophagy, as protein turnover typically lags with age even in the presence of excess growth signals. *A key gene in the autophagy process is the Target of Rapamycin (TAR)* and inhibition of this protein by the antibiotic Rapamycin has significantly extended lifespan in mice and other species. Likewise, inflammation results from chronic activation of compliment and other immune system genetic products (e.g. IL-6 and CRP). Finally, ion transport includes the genes involved with chloride, magnesium, and calcium transport, which are often imbalanced with age. Blood transport of lipids (ApoE, LDL, and HDL) is also very significant in the aging of the cardiovascular system.

The genetics of human longevity are still progressing rapidly with new genetic variants and pathways turning up on a regular basis. There is a continuously updated website on human longevity genetic pathways, which is available at http://genomics.senescence.info/longevity/.

In summary, it is very clear that aging has multiple causes and pathways that involve altered gene expression and many changes at both the cellular and systemic levels. Equally clear is the need for Multipath Rejuvenation (MuR) treatments to have a realistic chance of turning the aging body back toward a more youthful state.

9. Why We Age And Can It Be Controlled?

> "Aging occurs ... due to the declining forces of natural selection during adult life."
>
> **- Michael R. Rose**

Summary: Why we age and can it be controlled?

Aging is caused by the decline in the force of natural selection during adult life. While many aspects of fitness will naturally decline with adult age, Multipath Rejuvenation (MuR) treatments that correct many of the biological pathways responsible for the fitness decline may be able to regenerate much of the youthful fitness found in 30 to 40 year olds. Resetting the critical physiological markers of 40 to 65 year olds back to a stable fitness state of 30 to 40 year olds could potentially freeze the annual mortality rate at less than 0.2% and thereby greatly expand healthspan, lifespan, and youth.

In the previous chapter we discussed the many genes and genetic pathways that appear to be involved in the aging process. If you are confused by all this diverse genetic data on aging, you are not alone. It is difficult to come up with a simple view of the aging process given all the many genetic pathways that have been implicated in the process. As might be expected from the genetic research data, there are scores of theories on the causes of aging, which focus on one or more types of data or various genetic pathways. However, the typical theory of aging is often incomplete and only explains a fraction of the data. So how does one come up with a comprehensive concept of why aging occurs and its basic causes?

To begin the discussion about how most experts in the aging field think about why we age, we must go back to the basic Darwinian principle of **natural selection**. All life forms on earth have evolved through natural selection, which selects the best genotype for fitness in a particular ecological niche. In 1952 the British Nobel zoologist Peter Medawar proposed that ***aging is the simple result of the failure of natural selection to maintain fitness in older animals with declining fertility.*** As fertility wanes, then the chances to correct inappropriate gene expression via natural selection also decline, generating the aging phenotype. According to Medawar's hypothesis, ***aging is indirectly caused by the declining forces of natural selection to select the best fitness genes for the aged animal as reproduction capacity declines (Fig. 5). Thus, animal fitness levels will drop and mortality rates will increase as reproduction declines. Indeed, genetic selection against deleterious genes declines to zero post reproduction.***

In 1957, George Williams further developed Medawar's evolutionary theory of aging by introducing the concept of **antagonistic pleiotropy**, wherein a gene may promote fitness in young fertile animals (and thus be selected for) but become a liability late in life leading to a subsequent decline in fitness. Calcium binding proteins like the Matrix gla Proteins (MGPs) and osteocalcin are good examples of antagonistic pleiotropy. These calcium binding proteins promote rapid bone calcification in young growing animals, but can lead to slow calcification of blood vessels and organs in later adulthood as the calcium binding proteins decline in effectiveness.

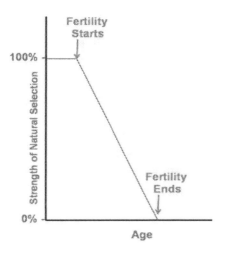

Fig. 5: **Strength of natural selection falls as reproduction declines.** Natural selection is the strongest before sexual maturity. As reproduction wanes, the strength of natural selection falls, so late-acting genetically unfit genes can accumulate.

Modern versions of Medawar's and William's evolutionary theories of aging are still widely believed today by most experts in aging science, as the theory fits well with the immense body of literature showing that natural selection is responsible for virtually all of the phenotypes present in the diverse species observed in Nature. Evolution appears to evolve a life history for each species that is best adapted to its ecological niche. For example, small land based rodents (e.g. mice and rats) typically have a short 2-3 year lifespan, as they are most often killed by predators before aging plays a major role in their mortality. In contrast, small flying animals (e.g. birds and bats) are much better protected from predators and have an extended innate lifespan of 15 to 30 years.

Besides its sound theoretical basis in the well-known mechanisms of natural selection, the Evolutionary Theory of Aging has also been directly tested in *Drosophila melanogaster* by Michael Rose at UCI. If the Evolutionary Theory of Aging was correct, Dr. Rose predicted that he should be able to select populations of long lived animals by simply selecting for reproductive longevity. To carry out his longevity experiment, Dr. Rose started with 5 lines of wild type *Drosophila* flies and selected for reproductive longevity over a 27 year period. Within a few years, Dr. Rose could tell that he was successfully generating longer living flies by selecting each fly generation for late fertility. He finally obtained robust Methuselah flies with a demonstrated lifespan of about 3 times that found in the non-selected control lines, while retaining fertility and sexual vitality. Genescient, Inc. (Irvine, CA) has carried out several independent experiments to verify that these Methuselah flies are indeed long lived compared to wild type flies. As Genescient's VP of R & D, I supervised the most recent comparative lifespan experiments on the Methuselah flies. As can be observed in Fig. 6 below, the Methuselah flies (O populations) far outlive their unselected wild type fly populations (B flies).

The results in Fig. 6 clearly demonstrate that it is straightforward to select for long-lived flies by selecting for delayed reproduction. A similar delayed reproduction selection has also been carried out on mice by the Canadian government. This mouse project was much more expensive than the fly research and had some unfortunate gaps in funding. While the mouse selection also appears to have resulted in significant gains in mouse longevity, these Methuselah mouse results have yet to be published in peer-reviewed journals because the project has remained incomplete due to funding issues.

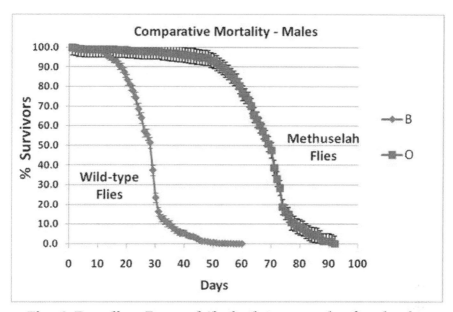

Fig. 6: Breeding *Drosophila* for late reproduction leads to much longer lived flies. O Methuselah flies live much longer than do Wild type B flies. The result is as predicted by the Evolution Theory of Aging.

A second line of evidence supporting the Evolutionary Theory of Aging is the prediction of the theory that the mortality rate should eventually plateau in late life due to the fact that reproduction and natural selection both decline to minimal levels or totally vanish in late life. The mortality rate likely continues to increase for some time post reproduction due to secondary network effects, which cause progressively more physiological disequilibrium at both the cell and organ level. Eventually these secondary effects would be exhausted and the theory predicts that the mortality rate will stabilize and plateau at some level short of 100%. This prediction is unique to the Evolutionary Theory of Aging, as aging is typically defined by an exponential increase in mortality rates until all of the population dies off. That mortality rates could actually plateau in late life was an unexpected finding that was only predicted by Dr. Rose using the Evolutionary Theory of Aging. Mortality rates have been shown to decelerate and then plateau in *Drosophila*, medflies, nematodes, wasps, and yeast (80-81).

While it is interesting that many model animals have a mortality rate plateau, the real question is does a mortality rate plateau also occur in humans? Humans have a typical exponential mortality rate curve up to about age 105 based on the Social Security Administration Death Master File containing millions of humans (see Fig. 7). Just like model organisms, the human mortality rate appears to flatten out eventually. Females undergo menopause at age 45 to 55, and the annual mortality rate appears to flatten out at around 107 to 110 years at an annual mortality rate of about 50% (bottom of Fig. 7).

While the data in Fig. 7 is very suggestive of a plateau in mortality rates at late ages, it is still questioned by some researchers because there are so few humans that have been validated to have lived 110 years or more. The data is particularly sparse for humans that have lived for over 116 years (very few humans have been validated to have lived 117 years or longer). Some have claimed that these long lived humans over 116 are merely outlier survivors. To my mind, this misses the point since all centenarians are outlier survivors in that they have escaped death from cardiovascular disease and cancer. That said, the data between 107 and 114 looks fairly robust, and it is clear that the existing data is not consistent with a continued exponential rise in annual mortality rates in the 107 to 120 age bracket. At the minimum, the exponential mortality rate increases appear to be suppressed after 107 years of age. As we have seen, this modulation in mortality is the expected result if the Evolutionary Theory of Aging is correct.

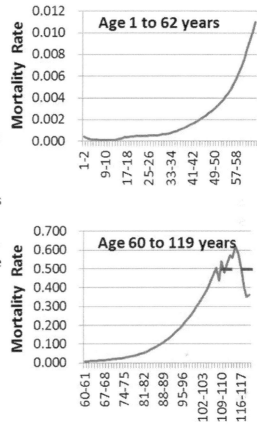

Fig. 7: Human annual mortality rate plateaus in late life. The rate of mortality is exponential from 25 to 107 years and then appears to plateau at about 50% mortality. All data under 110 years is from the Social Security Administration Death Master File, while 110 to 119 years is from validated human super-centenarians from www.grg.org .

Of course, this apparent plateau or slackening in growth of the annual mortality rate does not mean that aging has stopped or that individuals do not undergo further functional declines in the years after 107. Indeed, those over 107 face a minimum of 50-50 odds of dying for each and every year longer that they live. Those bleak annual survival odds are more like those of a terminal cancer patient than like individuals that have escaped the grim reaper.

Assuming there is a plateau or slowing of the rate of increase in the annual mortality rate after 107 years of age, the existence of a mortality rate plateau suggests that there may be a limited set of genetic pathways that are 'out of tune' at 50 to 55 years in humans, and that these pathways slowly generate a finite amount of future damage with age. The mortality rate is only 0.4% (4 per thousand people) per year at 55 (see top of Fig. 7).

If the unfit physiological patterns present at 55 years of age could be stabilized at this fitness state or better, we may be able to engineer the mortality rate to plateau at or below the 0.4% level, rather than the 50% plus level observed in centenarians of 107 and older. *The long term goal is to return the genetic pathways and the physiological fitness of 50 to 80 year olds to a more youthful state (say 30 to 40 years of age) and thereby to freeze the annual mortality rate at 0.1% to 0.2%. If we could accomplish this goal, human lifespan would be essentially indeterminate.* If we can significantly slow the increase in annual mortality rates by rebalancing or fine tuning our genetic expression (e.g. by using comprehensive MuR treatments), then average lifespan could be greatly expanded along with youth and fitness. Other future options for keeping the mortality rate from rising with age utilize regenerative stem cells or nanobots, as we will explore in the last chapter.

10. Cell Aging and Telomerase

"The cell, after all, is a machine, so why should it not simply wear out, just as an automobile does?"

- Albert Rosenfeld

Summary: Cell Aging and Telomerase

While embryonic stem cells are immortal, somatic cells and nearly all adult stem cells do senesce. Cell aging promotes cell dysfunction and aging. One of the major causes of cell aging is telomere loss, which starts in embryogenesis and continues throughout life. The enzyme telomerase can lengthen telomeres and reverse cell aging in many cells, but telomerase is turned off in most cells early in development. Treatments that activate telomerase can slow or reverse cell aging in many cell types, but is especially important in adult stem cells. Telomerase activation is likely most significant in delaying or reversing adult stem cell aging. However, telomere loss is not the only type of genetic damage that promotes cell aging. Limiting genomic, mitochondrial, and epigenetic damage can also slow the rate of cell aging.

The idea that the body just 'wears out' is an all-too-common belief about what causes aging. Aging is more complicated than the simple concepts of the accumulation of damage or of an aging body 'wearing out'. Indeed, the ever-popular *rate of living theory* of aging has been widely discredited by species comparison data. For example, bats are small animals with a fast metabolism like mice or rats and thus should have a similar lifespan according to the rate of living theory. Yet bats live 15 to 20 years while mice and rats typically live 2 to 3 years. Likewise, small birds live much longer than the rate of living theory would predict. In this chapter, we look at cells that senesce and immortal cancer and embryonic stem cells that do not senesce as further reasons to doubt the damage and rate of living theories.

Multicellular animals are typically composed of many tissues and organs, which can become dysfunctional by mechanical injury, infection, or age-related declines. But most tissues and organs also have the regenerative capacity to recover from damage or infection. For example, most cells have several systems to repair genetic damage, degrade damaged proteins, and make new proteins. Moreover, single-cell organisms that reproduce via the simple process of mitosis (splitting into two equal-sized cells) do not typically senesce. In most metastatic cancer lines and germ line stem cells from multicellular organism, cell metabolism and repair systems are so efficient that these cells are essentially immortal. In the case of cancer cells, the development of cell immortality is often an essential step to metastatic cancer. Germ line stem cells are also immortal as a cell reservoir of genetic information. Indeed, *your own germ line stem cells represent a continuous line of living cells going back to the original cells that started life billions of years ago!*

Excluding the immortal cells described above, there is some truth to the concept that normal *somatic cells* (i.e. cells that build body tissues other than the germ line stem cells) 'wear out' and senesce in that they have a finite capacity to divide, gradually lose critical functions, and eventually die. The aging of somatic cells is often termed **cell aging (or cell senescence)** and reflects the fact that normal human cells in cell culture can only divide about 40 to 70 divisions before reaching the aging limit. This cell division limit for non-cancer somatic cells was discovered in 1961 by Leonard Hayflick and has since been found to be a universal characteristic of normal human somatic cells. At the time, no one had a good explanation for why normal human cells had a limited capacity to divide while metastatic cancer cells could proliferate forever.

It was found in the early 1990s that each time normal human cells divide, they lose some telomere DNA at the ends of their chromosomes and it was suggested that *with the fully aged cell, telomere length becomes critically short, leading to cell dysfunction or death*. In contrast, telomere length in immortal cancer cells can vary in length, but does not typically shorten with division. This novel *Telomere Theory of Cell Aging* was testable if we could lengthen telomeres to see if this reversed cellular aging. Lengthening telomeres is possible if we activate telomerase, which is the enzyme responsible for adding telomeric DNA onto chromosome ends. The problem is *telomerase is turned off early in embryonic development* in most normal somatic cells, so that telomeres shorten with age in the typical somatic cell and can reach a critical shortened state (around 5,000 bases, see Fig. 8) wherein the cell is senescent and can no longer divide.

The mouse and human telomerase genes had not yet been identified in the early 1990s. In 1992 Michael West, who was then the CEO of Geron Corporation (a startup biotech company in Menlo Park, CA), visited me in my lab at the University of Michigan Institute of Gerontology to talk about his plans to make Geron the first biotech company to study aging using telomerase science. After that meeting I became very excited about telomerase and subsequently joined Geron in January of 1993 with the goal of cloning human telomerase. Several big academic groups had already been working on cloning telomerase from various species for years (e. g. Elizabeth Blackburn and Carol Greider, who won the 2009 Nobel Prize for their pioneering telomerase work), so Geron had obtained licensing contracts with them to help support the company's efforts to clone human telomerase. The RNA component of human telomerase was a particularly high value target and the academic labs did not welcome competition from Geron scientists in the actual discovery work. For a time, they were able to block Geron's internal research on cloning the human telomerase gene.

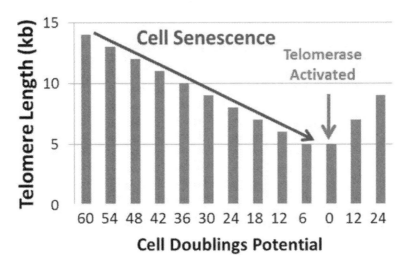

Cell Doublings Potential

Fig. 8: Telomeres shorten as cells senescence.
Telomeres shorten with cell division, leading to the loss of doubling capacity as well as loss of function. If telomerase is activated, telomeres can lengthen again to regenerate cell doubling potential and cell function.

By the fall of 1993, Geron scientists were finally given permission to identify and clone the human telomerase genes. In November of 1993, I devised a novel cyclic selection protocol for enriching the RNA component of human telomerase from normal lung fibroblasts. Candidate clones were selected by size and by their expression in telomerase positive cells versus non-expression in telomerase negative cells. By March of 1994, this experimental selection protocol successfully pulled out the RNA component of human telomerase. Verification of success took more than a year. In September 1995 a big article on the cloning of human telomerase was published in *Science* along with the cloning of the mouse RNA component (107-108). I subsequently led a team of about 25 scientists at Geron to clone the human protein component of telomerase. The team was finally successful in the spring of 1997. With the successful cloning of both the RNA and protein components of human telomerase, I subsequently left Geron in July of 1997 to join another new antiaging company in San Diego. Verification of the telomere theory of cellular aging came a year later when my scientific colleagues at Geron Corporation were able to use the cloned protein component of telomerase to demonstrate that *several types of normal somatic cells could be immortalized if genetically transformed to express high levels of the telomerase enzyme, adding back telomeric DNA to the shortened chromosome ends.*

In human development, telomerase is turned off in most somatic cells in the early embryo stage, which leads to telomere loss and a slower division potential as the cells reach a critically short telomere length. Telomerase-induced cell immortalization has since been repeated in many labs throughout the world and is now a well-established finding. Nevertheless, biology is complex and telomere loss is not the only cause of cell aging in some types of cells, so not all cell types are immortalized by telomerase. For example, the critical factor in keratinocytes aging is up-regulation of the p16 tumor suppressor gene.

The link of cellular aging and telomerase to human aging is controversial, but many of the scientists working on telomerase now believe that telomerase may play an important role in human aging. The ability of telomerase to immortalize normal fibroblasts led to the proposal that human aging might be slowed or partly reversed if one could activate telomerase to suppress cellular aging (109, 112). Several lines of evidence support this antiaging telomerase hypothesis. For example, telomeres tend to shorten in human lymphocytes extracted from volunteers as a function of age and those people with the shortest telomeres have increased risks of dying from age-related diseases. Another line of evidence came from experiments using senescent human fibroblasts that had been made immortal by telomerase expression and then surgically inserted on the back of mice to form mice with human skin. This 'telomerized' human skin was derived from senescent skin cells, but looked like young skin and had a similar profile of gene expression as did young skin. A third line of evidence comes from transgenic mice that had been engineered to over-express telomerase. These mice lived about one third longer when the innate defenses against cancer were also heightened.

A final line of evidence suggesting some antiaging effects of telomerase come from the limited human trials with a nutraceutical that very weakly activates telomerase activity. Geron Corporation collaborated with a Hong Kong company to identify telomerase activators in Chinese herbal medicines. The herbal telomerase-activators identified by this collaboration were the astragalosides and especially Astragaloside IV or its derivative cycloastragenol. Astragaloside IV is now widely believed to be a principle active agent in the Chinese herb known as *Astragalus membranaceus*. In short term (one year or less) clinical field trials with Astragaloside IV, investigators have reported increased energy, enhanced immunity, improved vision, and better skin condition. ***The above data suggests that telomerase activation might well help slow some aspects of the aging process, but it is unlikely to be very effective as a standalone treatment.***

Astragalus membranaceus herbal extracts have also been used in China for thousands of years as a tonic medicinal factor to combat cardiovascular and other disease states. But traditional medicinal use was often for less than one month duration. Thus, long term effects of treatment with *Astragalus* are not well documented.

Currently, the foremost company developing telomerase activators is **Sierra Sciences**, which is a Reno biotech company. Sierra Sciences has actually developed potent drugs functioning as telomerase activators, but as of this writing, all of the telomerase activating drugs have some cell toxicity and thus have not been tested in animals or humans. I have been on the Scientific Advisory board of Sierra Sciences since it was started in 1999 and have consulted extensively for the company. Although much of my time is now devoted to other pursuits, I am still interested in safe but potent telomerase activators when they become available. They may prove to be invaluable substances for helping to delay, stop, or even reverse the aging process. For the present, MuR supplements and lifestyle changes (see Chapters 4 to 6) are other options for maintaining one's telomeres.

Finally, one common criticism about the importance of cell aging and telomerase in aging should be addressed. Critics cite the fact that many of the most important adult human cell populations (e.g. neurons and muscle) do not divide and thus should not be affected by cell aging and telomere loss. But brain astrocytes are ten times more prevalent than neurons and provide critical support for neurons in the brain. Astrocytes are dividing cells with shortening telomeres. Also, there is the fact that neuronal and muscle tissue can be damaged with age, and must eventually be repaired and/or replaced. It has long been known that muscle satellite stem cells typically repair muscle tissue and it was recently found that adult neuronal stem cells also exist that can repair neuronal tissue. Indeed, adult neuronal and muscle stem cells are essential to the full repair of both neurons and muscle.

Unfortunately, **adult stem cell populations and/or their immediate environment decline significantly with age, which is likely due to cell aging of a fraction of the cells.** While few studies have looked at telomere loss in neuronal and muscle stem cells, telomere loss has been observed with age in the case of hematopoietic stem cells and has led to fewer functional lymphocytes and inferior immune response.

As previously mentioned, telomere loss is not the only cause of cellular aging. Examples of other factors linked to cellular aging include: accumulation of the p16 gene product, genomic DNA damage, epigenetic alteration of histones, and a loss of mitochondrial DNA sequences or structure. All of the causes of cell aging need to be addressed if we want to limit aging of our stem cells, which are critical to regeneration of organs and tissues damaged by disease, injury, or aging. Moreover, cell turnover and the removal of functionally old cells is a critical factor, as senescent cells excrete toxic or damaging molecules that compromise healthy surrounding tissue and can cause systemic damage.

11. The Cardiovascular System

"A man is as old as his arteries."

- Thomas Sydenhan

Summary: The Cardiovascular system

Preservation of the vascular system is critical to extending lifespan. The vascular system of arteries, veins, and capillaries maintains the microenvironment around cells. With age the vascular system declines with about half of the capillaries vanishing in later years. This affects every organ in the body, leaving the cells starved for nutrients and oxygen, and spawning aberrant cell growth and fibrosis. This must be controlled to reverse functional decline with age. The lymphatic system is an independent system of circulation that also needs to be maintained to rid the body of waste.

The main age-related changes to the vascular system include *atherosclerosis* (buildup of plaques in the lumen of arteries), *arteriosclerosis* (the loss of elasticity and calcification of the arteries), vein stiffening, and loss of many small capillaries that feed organs and tissues. All of these changes promote increases in blood pressure with age and the reduction in blood circulation to vital organs and tissues. *Atherosclerosis is the global basis of most mortality in humans*, which often presents as failure in critical organs such as the heart, brain, or kidneys.

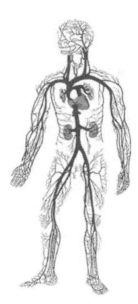

The heart is the most obvious example of a vital organ that is critical to life and death. Although myocardial (heart) cells do accumulate lipofuscin and there can be changes in ventricle wall thickness and the calcification of heart valves with age, heart disease is predominantly the result of the decline or catastrophic failure in the cardiac vascular system that feeds the heart. Current treatments for heart disease use this understanding to prevent or slow the progression of heart disease by controlling blood pressure, blood lipids, and chronic inflammation, which are all key factors in promoting atherosclerosis.

Besides the heart, atherosclerosis also causes damage to other critical organs such as the brain, kidneys, liver, skin, skeletal muscle, intestines, and various glands. The large human brain is very active and uses a lot of oxygen and only works on glucose as an energy source (unlike most other organs and tissues). This makes it hyper sensitive to vascular failure, which presents as major or minor strokes. Vascular failure in the brain leads to strokes that kill neurons, which cannot be regenerated because of the very low numbers of neural stem cell populations.

Another major killer is end-stage renal disease (kidney failure). With the reduced circulation to the kidney, kidney structure and function declines, which leads to a failure to remove many toxins and waste products from the blood. If end-stage renal failure is not treated with a successful kidney transplant or with continual kidney machine dialysis, death ensues. Normal aging typically leads to significant declines in kidney function and less than optimal removal of waste products in the blood. Optimal cell microenvironment is heavily dependent on fully functioning kidneys.

Peripheral Arterial Disease (PAD) is a common nonlethal condition caused by atherosclerosis. Skeletal muscles in the extremities are most affected by PAD, as capillary density to the arms and legs is reduced. Although without symptoms in the early stages of the disease, PAD can eventually lead to muscle pain or cramping while exercising (intermittent claudication). In chronic conditions of PAD, affected individual can also experience numbness, weakness, atrophy, paleness, hair loss, and/or poor wound healing due to poor circulation to their extremities. While only a proportion of people will experience the worst complication of PAD, loss of capillaries and reduced blood circulation are typical conditions with advancing age in the extremities. And reduced circulation does have adverse effects on the microenvironment around cells.

Any discussion of the body's circulatory system should include the lymphatic system. The cardiovascular system is responsible for distributing oxygen, nutrients, and hormones, and for removing metabolic waste products. The lymphatic system is a secondary circulatory system that removes other types of waste (infectious agents, old blood cells, and toxic waste from the interstitial fluid) and provides a reservoir of new blood cells. Note that the lymphatic circulation is a passive flow system with one-way valves that is dependent on muscle movement. Thus, *activities like stretching, deep breathing, and frequent exercise are all essential for maintaining optimal circulation in the lymphatic system.* While blood is filtered by the kidneys, the lymphatic system is filtered by the lymph nodes, which can remove pathogens, cell debris, cancers, and toxins. Obviously, a well-working lymphatic system is essential for improving healthspan and longevity.

In conclusion, the decline of the vasculature strongly promotes major organ decline. Not only do clogged and calcified blood vessels starve organs of oxygen and food, but *poorly functioning vasculature promotes organ microenvironments where abnormal cells, fibrosis, and inappropriate calcification are promoted in all the major organs. Organ dysfunctions (especially in the lungs, intestines, liver, and kidneys) then cause further deterioration in the vasculature and organ systems in a downward spiral.*

12. Nervous System and Sensory Organs

> "All diseases run into one, old age."

> **- Ralph Waldo Emerson**

Summary: Nervous System and Sensory Organs

The main initiators of brain aging are the general decay in the micro-environment, which includes chronic inflammation, toxin buildup, altered metabolism, and decline in vascular supply. Inside neurons, both the buildup of damaged proteins (e.g. tau tangles and beta-amyloid) and alteration in the pattern of gene expression also play key roles. The end result may be neuronal loss, but the most significant initial losses are the regression in axon connectivity as the density of dendritic arbors and spines declines.

The nervous system is composed of an interconnected network of neural cells that is divided into the *central nervous system* (brain and spinal cord) and the *peripheral nervous system* (sensory neurons, ganglia clusters, and connecting nerves). Neural cells include the **neurons** and the tenfold more abundant **glial cells**, wherein glia are further divided into astrocytes, oligodendrocytes, and microglia. Neurons are believed to play a major role in memory and motor function, while glial cells play an important metabolic support function to the neurons.

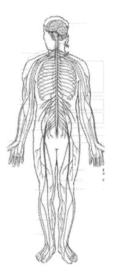

Brain aging is often observed as cognitive decline, which is linked to loss of vascular supply and instabilities in the microenvironment around neurons. In Chapter 11 above we discussed the decline of vascular supply in the heart, brain, and other critical organs. As is well known, sudden loss of blood circulation to part of the brain can lead to both major and minor strokes. But even if strokes are avoided, there is often a gradual decline of vascular supply to the brain with age. Changes in vascular supply and inflammation then lead to a *dysfunctional microenvironment around neurons in the brain*, which can lead to age-related cognitive decline. If the neural changes are severe enough, then you end up with pathologies like Alzheimer's disease or vascular dementia.

With its billions of neurons and thousands of connections for each neuron, *the neural network is very dependent on its vascular supply, glial helper cells, and the larger micro-environment for optimal function.* The changes in general micro-environment with age include: increased cerebral perfusion pressure, toxin buildup, amyloid plaque, chronic inflammation, and altered hormonal balance. On average, the brain loses about 5 to 10% of its weight from the early 20s to the 90s. *Significantly, the dendrites and dentritic spines that connect neurons to each other (i.e. brain wiring) also decline with age.* Inside neurons, the number of *neurofibriallary tangles (tau)*, which are twisted protein fiber aggregates, also increases with advancing age, limiting the arbor growth and spine connection.

For a generation, the conventional wisdom was that neuronal loss and amyloid plaque were driving age-related cognitive decline and Alzheimer's disease. In the last few years, this conventional wisdom has been challenged by the fact that many elderly people are found to have amyloid plaque without any signs of cognitive decline or Alzheimer's disease. Conversely, some Alzheimer's disease patients appear to have little amyloid plaque. Even more destructive to the amyloid plaque theory, clinical trials have indicated that beta-amyloid reduction appears to have a neutral or even negative effects on Alzheimer's patients. While amyloid plaque appears to be one of the causes of cognitive decline, other factors must also play a prominent role.

If amyloid plaque is not the prime cause of dementia and age-related functional decline, then what is? Besides changes within the central part of the brain neurons themselves (e.g. changes in gene expression, mitochondrial dysfunction, oxidized protein aggregates, and tangled fibers), *there is also a marked reduction in dentritic spine number and dentritic density along with a general decay of the myelin sheath covering neuronal axons (82-86)*. These neuronal changes lead to a decline of neuron to neuron communication and axon connectivity. Given that each neuron has more than a thousand connections to other neurons to encode memory and behavior, the general decline in neuron to neuron connections naturally leads to brain network disruptions and cognitive decline.

13. Indefinite Healthspans by 2050?

> "The idea is to die young as late as possible."

> **- Ashley Montagu**

Summary: Indefinite Healthspans by 2050?

The rate of technology advancement has been accelerating in an exponential progression for at least the last 75 years and appears poised to keep on its exponential path for at least another 50 years. This exponential rate of technological change has impacted humans in every aspect of life and shows every indication of moving ever faster for the foreseeable future. In particular, mean life expectancy has increased annually for over 110 years as modern technology has been employed. Projecting these historical and exponential trends onto the next 40 years, one optimistic prediction is that by 2050 the annual incremental increases in life expectancy will have reached the *"Longevity Escape Velocity"*, where advancing technology adds a year of healthspan and lifespan for every year that you live.

Even in this optimistic projection, humans would still be far from immortal, as many will still die from accidents or disease or poor lifestyle choices. For example, some forms of cancer, dementia, viral infections, or substance abuse may not be effectively treated even with the formable tools available by the mid-21st Century.

Even with people still dying from multiple causes in 2050, age may not be the major factor in mortality risks as it is today. For example, the annual risk of dying normally increases with age with the risk of all-cause mortality doubling every 8 years after age 25. The accumulated technology available by 2050 should greatly slow or even stop this rise in mortality risks with age. In this case, the firm expectation is that health and fitness will also slow its decline with age or may even stop declining at some age. This will greatly increase healthspan and fitness in the over 60 population, so getting older would lose much or all of its negative aspects. Indeed, *expanding healthspan and fitness is the ultimate goal, as lifespan gains without concurrent advances in health and youthful fitness would not be viewed as beneficial by most people.*

The table below is my best guess on the future strategies and technologies that will increase healthspan and lifespan. Notice that healthspan is typically projected to increase more than lifespan.

Strategy/Technology	When Available	Healthspan Extension	Lifespan Extension
Diet and Nutrition	Now	10-35	2-15
Regular Moderate Exercise	Now	5-20	2-10
Dietary Supplements	2013-2050	3-30 (?)	2-20 (?)
Hormones	2013-2020	1-5 (?)	1-2 (?)
Drugs	2013-2050	3-30 (?)	2-20 (?)
Stem Cells	2013-2025	2-80 (?)	2-40 (?)
Organ Regeneration	2013-2040	5-100 (?)	2-50 (?)
Nano Technology	2020-2050	5-150 (?)	5-150 (?)

Near Term Technologies for Extending Healthspan

The first five rows of the above table give a good summary of the technologies available today to extend healthspan and lifespan (diet, exercise, some dietary supplements, hormones, and a few drugs). Of course, diet and exercise are the furthest along, while much more research and development will be required for supplements, hormones, and drugs to reach their optimal potential.

A few Vitamin and mineral ***dietary supplements*** have been linked to longevity: ***Vitamin D3*** (87-89, 91), ***Vitamin K*** (90), ***magnesium*** (92-95), ***selenium*** (96-98), and ***lithium*** (99-101).   Our group at Genescient has shown that the complex herbal product SC100 greatly extends the healthspan and lifespan of Drosophila (unpublished data). A small human field trial indicated that SC100 lowered blood pressure, glucose, and lipids, suggesting that human healthspan could also be extended.   We have recently improved on the SC100 formulation with a new composition Memex 100™ that adds comprehensive neural protection. A clinical trial on Memex 100™ was started in October, 2013. It is a safe prediction that there will be many other dietary supplements and drugs that will be found to extend healthspan and lifespan in the coming decades.

Treatment with ***hormones*** is still controversial as to efficacy in extending healthspan except in the case of insulin for diabetics and perhaps estrogen for post-menopausal women. The case for growth hormone or testosterone is more complicated, as there are clear short-term benefits paired with potential harm in the long term. But we may see new hormone treatments in the next 10 to 20 years that overcome some of the current difficulties and are proven to extend healthspan and perhaps life expectancy.

Drugs are another strategy for extending both healthspan and lifespan, as new longevity gene targets are now being found at a rapid rate, while a large number of longevity genes have already been identified. Of the current drugs that are available on the market and relatively safe to take, ***low-dose aspirin*** (102-105) and the ***statin drugs*** (106) have been shown to lower all-cause mortality and morbidity, which is a strong marker of antiaging potential. Of course, statins can have serious side effects, so statin drugs are best used at the lowest doses, while relying on diet, exercise, and supplements to do the major work of lowering cholesterol. Other potential antiaging drugs in the near term are rapamycin and its analogs, which target autophagy, and drugs that target growth hormone or growth hormone receptors.

Unfortunately, the potential opportunities for antiaging drugs are limited in that aging uses multiple pathways rather than the single pathway targeting favored by drug companies and the FDA. Moreover, the FDA does not have a regulatory path for approving an antiaging drug, so any potential antiaging drug would have to get regulatory approval as a cure or preventive for an age-related disease indication rather than the aging process itself. Because of the pharmaceutical focus on single compounds and the difficulties of FDA compliance rules, complex dietary supplements with many components acting on multiple synergistic pathways are much less costly to develop and more likely to be effective as longevity treatments than single component pharmaceuticals. That was our principle in developing SC100 and Memex 100™.

Stem Cells and Organ Regeneration

The best hope for dramatic increases in healthspan and lifespan in the next 10 to 20 years comes from the use of **stem cells** for systemic effects in the body, tissue regeneration *in vivo*, and **organ regeneration** in lab incubators. Currently most researchers in the stem cell field are working with **Embryonic Stem (ES)** cells or **induced Pluripotent Stem (iPS)** cells. There are significant problems with utilizing ES cell lines as a universal donor. First, there is the problem of potential immune system reaction when foreign cells are introduced into the body. Many proponents say that ES cell lines do not elicit host immune response, but the long term effects on immune response have not been tested. Second, there are ethical issues involved with the sacrifice of human embryos to produce the ES cells, which has limited the research and development of ES lines. Third, it is not easy to derive the specialized cells needed using ES cells. Fourth, ES cells can produce teratomas (germ line cancer cells) and even a small risk of cancer is a major safety concern.

The most exciting scientific discovery in the stem cell field in the last decade is that normal adult skin cells can be converted into embryonic-like stem cells (called **iPS cells** for induced-pluripotent stem cells) by the expression of only four genes: Oct4, Sox2, c-myc, and Kf4. The iPS cells can be derived from your own cells, so the first two potential problems with ES cells are solved using iPS cells. However, the iPS technology typically uses genetic manipulation to insert Oct4, Sox2, c-myc, and Kf4 into a patient's skin cell line to generate the iPS cells, which can lead to the potential of activating cancer genes. Moreover, to the extent that the iPS cells fully revert to the embryonic state (which is often not the case due to epigenetic factors), the resulting iPS cells often have difficulty efficiently forming some specialized tissues and organs. Therefore, the use of iPS cells in regenerative therapy may take a decade or more of further development before widespread use in the clinic. However, recent published papers have successfully created iPS cells using drugs instead of genetic methods, which could speed up the use of iPS in humans.

The third developing technology uses a patient's own **Adult Stem (AS)** cells found in the patient's bone marrow, fat deposits, or blood. The natural role of AS cells is to repair injured tissues and organs. AS cells do not have any of the drawbacks of ES or iPS cells, so virtually all of the stem cell treatments being done presently have been carried out using AS cells from bone marrow or belly fat or unbiblical cord blood.

Recently, there have been reports that even older people have a few AS cells that are apparently pluripotent. Pluripotency is the ability of a stem cell to form all three embryonic-like tissue layers (endodermal, mesodermal, and ectodermal) and through them any of the many specialized cells in the body. Conventional wisdom has been that only embryonic stem cells from the embryo or iPS cells were pluripotent enough to form all tissues, while adult stem cells were at best multipotent and could only form a limited number of specialized cells. Several papers have challenged that view by characterizing adult "Muse" and VSEL stem cells that appear to be pluripotent and embryo like. I call them **Adult Pluripotent Stem (APS)** cells.

The existence of these adult pluripotent stem (APS) cells has not been validated by some investigators, so there is still controversy as to their existence or prevalence. If APS cells do exist, the main problem may be that there are so few

APS cells in the adult (far fewer than 1% of AS cells are likely APS cells), which makes it a challenge to isolate enough cells from a patient's bone marrow or fat tissue to study. Moreover, growing the rare APS cells to get enough cells for analysis or clinical use presents another challenge, as the pluripotent nature can be easily lost if the cells are not handled or grown properly.

If one could expand APS cells a million fold without aging or changing their pluripotent ability to form all tissue types, the hope is that a large number of vibrant young APS cells could be injected back into your body after injury or disease to regenerate your senescing cells. In this case, many organ systems in the elderly could be rejuvenated. Expanding APS cells without aging or loss of pluripotency is exactly the game-changing technology that could really make giant strides in expanding human lifespan. No genetic engineering of the stem cells needs to take place with APS cells. Thus, APS expansion is inherently much safer and less risky than the ES or iPS technologies that most stem cell companies are pursuing. It is for this reason that I cofounded an adult stem cell company *Centagen* (see www.Centagen.com) to help develop APS cell technology. If APS cells do not actually exist, the technology to expand Adult Multipotent Stem (AMS) cells without aging them or limiting their multipotent potential could also be of great utility in clinical applications.

Whichever technology wins out, it is clear that young vigorous ES, iPS, APS, AMS cells will eventually transform medicine and provide a powerful tool to regenerate most or all tissue in the body. While no one can be certain that stem cells will act to counteract most or all of the declines in cell and tissue structures that characterizes aging (the aging brain and spinal cord may present particularly difficult targets), the evolving stem cell revolution certainly has the potential to extend lifespan much further than any previous medical or biotech technology.

Organ Regeneration is a further game-changing technology that is related to and typically based on stem cell biology. Using any of the pluripotent stem cells mentioned above or even multipotent cells (e.g. mesenchymal stem cells), it is now possible to grow whole organs in the lab. One way to do this is to use a synthetic scaffold and put in multipotent or pluripotent stem cells to grow the organ in all three dimensions. Simple organs such as ears, skin, blood vessels, wind pipes, and bladders have already been successfully grown in the lab. Many patients have already received a transplant of one of these simple lab-grown organs and are functioning well with them.

Of course, more complicated organs such as kidney, liver, and the heart are much more difficult to grow in the lab, but dramatic progress is being made here as well. One pioneer in the field is Dr. Anthony Attala of the Wake Forest Institute for Regenerative Medicine (WFIRM) in Winston-Salem, North Carolina. Dr. Attala has made ears and bladders for several years and is now making many more organs, including engineering liver tissue and ***3D printing of human kidneys*** (e.g. see Dr. Attala's technology in this video at http://www.youtube.com/watch?v=bX3C20104MA). Dr. Attala and other workers at WFIRM are now working on more than 30 different organs and tissues.

Besides the 3D printing of organs, another striking breakthrough in building complicated organs like the heart was the discovery that one could take an existing heart and enzymatically digest away all of the living cells leaving only the collagen and extracellular matrix of the heart. This "ghost" heart matrix was then seeded with new animal stem cells that grew on the existing matrix to produce a young regenerated organ populated with only the animal's own cells. This has actually been done with rat hearts and it forms a functioning beating heart!

Of course, it is still early in organ regeneration, so we cannot be sure what the final organ regeneration technology will entail. But it is a near certain bet that 3D printing is going to be a big part of the technology based on the known ability of 3D printing to print stem cells and all the differing types of organ matrix material, while permitting everything to be carried out in a precisely controlled sterile process.

For a historic perspective of organ regeneration, you could view the 3D stem cell printing of organs and tissue structures as analogous to the creation of the printed integrated circuits in electronics. In addition, the 3D printing technology that is used to print whole organs is enabled by the technological gains in stem cell biology, which is analogous to the invention of the transistor in electronics. Recall that the transistor and the printed integrated circuits powered the information and computer revolutions of the last 40 years. Likewise, stem cell technology and the 3D printing of stem cell networks will enable the creation of organs and spare body parts on demand.

If one needs a new liver, lung, heart, kidney, leg, or arm, fully functional tissues and organs made with rejuvenated stem cells should be relatively easy to produce within the next 10 to 25 years. That means that no one should die of a heart attack or kidney failure or type I diabetes. Moreover, if one adds periodic intravenous injections of hundreds of millions of rejuvenating stem cells that can renovate your circulatory system and do many systemic repairs to organs and tissues throughout the body, it is not difficult to envision significant increases in expected lifespans for those undergoing these regenerative organ and stem cell treatments.

If you are thinking about who will be able to afford these kinds of high tech organ and stem cell treatments, it is already the case that current stem cell treatments of injured knees using non-optimized adult stem cells from adipose tissue typically cost much less than standard knee reconstruction surgery. Yet, stem cell therapies appear to last much longer with less pain and down time when compared to standard treatments.

Nanotechnology and Bionic Tissues

To understand the potential for human life extension with nanotechnology, it is helpful to recall some recent technological history in the non-biological field of electronics. In the 1950s, computers with memories more than a million times smaller than that found in today's smart phones filled a medium-sized room and several technicians were required to keep the computer running. Practically no one predicted in the 50s or 60s that reliable personal computers with very large memories would be cheap and available to all, as they were by the 1990s. The same is true for internet access, which 25 years ago was limited to a few hundred scientists exchanging data files. And as with computers and the internet, who could have predicted 20 years ago that most people would own powerful and inexpensive mobile phones by 2010? Today, your cell phone has a million times more processing power than did the large room-sized IBM computer of the 1950s and costs more than ten thousand times less.

What powered all of these technological revolutions was the invention of the transistor and printed integrated circuits. With the invention of tiny transistor-powered chips, **Moore's Law** took effect, wherein the number of transistors that can be placed on small integrated circuits doubles at an exponential rate every two years. Despite many predictions of its imminent demise, Moore's Law is still projected to hold steady for many more years. It has strongly accelerated biological and genetic research, as it has all other sciences, and will likely continue to do so for the next few decades.

The first draft of a human genome was sequenced by the year 2000 at a cost of nearly $2 billion. The cost to sequence a human genome 10 years later in 2010 was about $50,000 and that price is expected to drop to $1000 by 2015. While inexpensive genome sequencing has been a boon to basic biological sciences including aging research, it has not led to many human disease cures as originally predicted. However, this is likely to change rapidly once the price of human genome sequencing falls to $1,000 or less. When millions of people have had their DNA sequenced, we will learn much more about the role of genetics in aging and disease. Likewise, the costs of gene expression profiling are also falling rapidly, which means that getting reliable data about how people genetically respond to aging, disease, or therapeutic treatments will increase tremendously in the coming decades, leading to many more viable treatments for human health and fitness with age. Since aging is a multipath process involving scores of genes, the genomic revolution still has the potential to generate new longevity gene targets and potential treatments.

Empowered by ever more sophisticated and sensitive electronic equipment, biological research itself is still expanding at an exponential rate. This has led to a biotech boom starting in the late 70s that clearly mimics the electronic revolution of the last 60 years. Not only are we learning much more about how cells, organs, and biological systems work, but we are now learning to regenerate tissues and organs using stem cells as described above.

A more direct linking of the electronic and biological revolutions is now seen in the first **bionic organs** (e.g. see http://www.extremetech.com/extreme/154893-researchers-create-worlds-first-3d-printed-bionic-organ As 3D printing of biological structures become more routine, 3D printing of electronic structures is also making huge gains. The first successful combination of these two revolutionary technologies has recently been described by a group at Princeton University in New Jersey. The researchers printed out an ear-like organ that has a hydrogel matrix material with an embedded coiled antenna printed with silver nanoparticles. In testing such devices, these Princeton researchers were able to detect radio waves in stereo using two bionic ears.

The next obvious step is to print nerve cells into the matrix material to have a direct connection to a coiled antenna or a microprocessor chip. As cell printing advances to finer scales using 3D micro-droplet printing, printed stem cells could evolve very close interfaces with nano-electronic devices that enable reliable sensors to be produced. With technology like this being developed, can an implanted brain sensor for Wi-Fi transmission be that distant in the future?

Nano robotics is an emerging technology with the goal of creating tiny robotic machines that are 0.1 to 10 microns in size. The larger 7 to 8 micron sizes are very close to the size of small stem cells and human red blood cells (RBCs). Human cells typically range in size from 7 to 100 microns, so nano-scale biotech robotic products ("**biobots**") could be made in a range of sizes and still be injectable through a small 25 gauge needle. Once nano 3D printers are able to print in the sub-micron scale, biobots of 8 to 100 microns could be produced at acceptable cost. Sensory biobots could be specially designed to easily interface with neurons if they are serving as sensors. These biobots could then be printed along with stem cells to form truly integrated **bionic sensors** and other **bionic tissues** with superhuman capabilities. Note that many biobots will likely be made out of biodegradable material, so they can be broken down by the body when no longer needed or they can move to a certain region of the body to be removed manually. Moreover, perhaps the optimal biobots will be *self-replicating synthetic cells*, which are currently under development by Craig Venter – see http://www.newscientist.com/article/dn23266-craig-venter-close-to-creating-synthetic-life.html#.UiyLUDYqjwE. The self-replicating aspects of synthetic cells could be designed to only be active outside the body, so the cell dose in the body is fully determined by the injected cell number.

Even before bionic tissues are created, small 7 micron biobots may be injected into the circulation system. These circulating biobots certainly could be very helpful for diagnostics (with attached sensors), tissue repair, drug or peptide dispensers, detox agents, or search and destroy (against cancer cells or infectious agents). Some diagnostic biobots are already in development.

While biobots are currently in the very early stages of development, it is easy to see that biobots could become powerful tools in disease management, tissue repair, and extending both healthspan and longevity.

The multiple factors driving the exponential rise in the risks of mortality and morbidity with age are embedded in our biology and genetics. It will not be easy to change this trajectory, but the exponential improvements in the technologies described above provide a strong basis for the prediction that most diseases will be cured and aging rate slowed or stopped in the next 40 years. The first and most important changes will be the extension of human healthspan. Lifespan will also increase as a side effect of improved healthspan and fitness, because mortality (death) and morbidity (health) are strongly linked to the aging process. As the antiaging technologies come on line, the linkage of age to mortality and morbidity will be weakened or obliterated. That means we can all have longer healthier lives with more time to enjoy the world, our friends, and our families.

References

1.   **Aigaki T, Seong KH, and Matsuo T**. Longevity determination genes in Drosophila melanogaster. *Mech Ageing Dev* 123: 1531-1541, 2002.

2.   **Ames BN**. Delaying the mitochondrial decay of aging. *Ann N Y Acad Sci* 1019: 406-411, 2004.

3.   **Andziak B, O'Connor TP, and Buffenstein R**. Antioxidants do not explain the disparate longevity between mice and the longest-living rodent, the naked mole-rat. *Mech Ageing Dev* 126: 1206-1212, 2005.

4.   **Anselmi CV, Malovini A, Roncarati R, Novelli V, Villa F, Condorelli G, Bellazzi R, and Puca AA**. Association of the FOXO3A locus with extreme longevity in a southern Italian centenarian study. *Rejuvenation Res* 12: 95-104, 2009.

5.   **Bartke A**. New findings in gene knockout, mutant and transgenic mice. *Exp Gerontol* 43: 11-14, 2008.

6.   **Bartke A, and Brown-Borg H**. Life extension in the dwarf mouse. *Curr Top Dev Biol* 63: 189-225, 2004.

7.   **Blair SN, Cheng Y, and Holder JS**. Is physical activity or physical fitness more important in defining health benefits? *Med Sci Sports Exerc* 33: S379-399; discussion S419-320, 2001.

8.   **Blasco MA**. Telomere length, stem cells and aging. *Nat Chem Biol* 3: 640-649, 2007.

9.   **Blasco MA, Funk W, Villeponteau B, and Greider CW**. Functional characterization and developmental regulation of mouse telomerase RNA. *Science* 269: 1267-1270, 1995.

10.   **Bond J, Jones C, Haughton M, DeMicco C, Kipling D, and Wynford-Thomas D**. Direct evidence from siRNA-directed "knock down" that p16(INK4a) is required for human fibroblast senescence and for limiting ras-induced epithelial cell proliferation. *Exp Cell Res* 292: 151-156, 2004.

11.   **Brookes S, Rowe J, Gutierrez Del Arroyo A, Bond J, and Peters G**. Contribution of p16(INK4a) to replicative

senescence of human fibroblasts. *Exp Cell Res* 298: 549-559, 2004.

12.   **Buchman AS, Boyle PA, Wilson RS, Bienias JL, and Bennett DA**. Physical activity and motor decline in older persons. *Muscle Nerve* 35: 354-362, 2007.

13.   **Burgering BM, and Kops GJ**. Cell cycle and death control: long live Forkheads. *Trends Biochem Sci* 27: 352-360, 2002.

14.   **Chandrashekar V, Dawson CR, Martin ER, Rocha JS, Bartke A, and Kopchick JJ**. Age-related alterations in pituitary and testicular functions in long-lived growth hormone receptor gene-disrupted mice. *Endocrinology* 148: 6019-6025, 2007.

15.   **Chen D, Pan KZ, Palter JE, and Kapahi P**. Longevity determined by developmental arrest genes in Caenorhabditis elegans. *Aging Cell* 6: 525-533, 2007.

16.   **Cho E, Seddon JM, Rosner B, Willett WC, and Hankinson SE**. Prospective study of intake of fruits, vegetables, Vitamins, and carotenoids and risk of age-related maculopathy. *Arch Ophthalmol* 122: 883-892, 2004.

17.   **Cowen T**. A heady message for lifespan regulation. *Trends Genet* 17: 109-113, 2001.

18.   **Crouch PJ, Cimdins K, Duce JA, Bush AI, and Trounce IA**. Mitochondria in aging and Alzheimer's disease. *Rejuvenation Res* 10: 349-357, 2007.

19.   **Dorman JB, Albinder B, Shroyer T, and Kenyon C**. The age-1 and daf-2 genes function in a common pathway to control the lifespan of Caenorhabditis elegans. *Genetics* 141: 1399-1406, 1995.

20.   **Epel ES, Lin J, Wilhelm FH, Wolkowitz OM, Cawthon R, Adler NE, Dolbier C, Mendes WB, and Blackburn EH**. Cell aging in relation to stress arousal and cardiovascular disease risk factors. *Psychoneuroendocrinology* 31: 277-287, 2006.

21.   **Feng J, Funk WD, Wang SS, Weinrich SL, Avilion AA, Chiu CP, Adams RR, Chang E, Allsopp RC, and Villeponteau B**. The RNA component of human telomerase. *Science* 269: 1236-1241, 1995.

22.   **Fielding J, Husten C, and Eriksen M**. Tobacco: Health Effects and Control. In: *Public Health and Preventive Medicine*, edited by Maxcy K, Rosenau M, Last J, Wallace R, and BN D. New York: McGraw Hill, 1998, p. 817–845.

23.   **Flachsbart F, Caliebe A, Kleindorp R, Blanche H, von Eller-Eberstein H, Nikolaus S, Schreiber S, and Nebel A**. Association of FOXO3A variation with human longevity confirmed in German centenarians. *Proc Natl Acad Sci U S A* 106: 2700-2705, 2009.

24.   **Flurkey K, Papaconstantinou J, Miller RA, and Harrison DE**. Lifespan extension and delayed immune and collagen aging in mutant mice with defects in growth hormone production. *Proc Natl Acad Sci U S A* 98: 6736-6741, 2001.

25.   **Garofalo RS**. Genetic analysis of insulin signaling in Drosophila. *Trends Endocrinol Metab* 13: 156-162, 2002.

26.   **Geserick C, and Blasco MA**. Novel roles for telomerase in aging. *Mech Ageing Dev* 127: 579-583, 2006.

27.   **Giannakou ME, and Partridge L**. Role of insulin-like signalling in Drosophila lifespan. *Trends Biochem Sci* 32: 180-188, 2007.

28.   **Hagen TM, Yowe DL, Bartholomew JC, Wehr CM, Do KL, Park JY, and Ames BN**. Mitochondrial decay in hepatocytes from old rats: membrane potential declines, heterogeneity and oxidants increase. *Proc Natl Acad Sci U S A* 94: 3064-3069, 1997.

29.   **Hamilton B, Dong Y, Shindo M, Liu W, Odell I, Ruvkun G, and Lee SS**. A systematic RNAi screen for longevity genes in C. elegans. *Genes Dev* 19: 1544-1555, 2005.

30.   **Harley CB**. Telomerase therapeutics for degenerative diseases. *Curr Mol Med* 5: 205-211, 2005.

31.   **Harley CB, and Villeponteau B**. Telomeres and telomerase in aging and cancer. *Curr Opin Genet Dev* 5: 249-255, 1995.

32.   **Holzenberger M**. The GH/IGF-I axis and longevity. *Eur J Endocrinol* 151 Suppl 1: S23-27, 2004.

33.   **Holzenberger M, Dupont J, Ducos B, Leneuve P, Geloen A, Even PC, Cervera P, and Le Bouc Y**. IGF-1

receptor regulates lifespan and resistance to oxidative stress in mice. *Nature* 421: 182-187, 2003.

34.   **Honda Y, and Honda S**. Oxidative stress and life span determination in the nematode Caenorhabditis elegans. *Ann N Y Acad Sci* 959: 466-474, 2002.

35.   **Hu G, Jousilahti P, Barengo NC, Qiao Q, Lakka TA, and Tuomilehto J**. Physical activity, cardiovascular risk factors, and mortality among Finnish adults with diabetes. *Diabetes Care* 28: 799-805, 2005.

36.   **Hudson EK, Hogue BA, Souza-Pinto NC, Croteau DL, Anson RM, Bohr VA, and Hansford RG**. Age-associated change in mitochondrial DNA damage. *Free Radic Res* 29: 573-579, 1998.

37.   **Hung HC, Joshipura KJ, Jiang R, Hu FB, Hunter D, Smith-Warner SA, Colditz GA, Rosner B, Spiegelman D, and Willett WC**. Fruit and vegetable intake and risk of major chronic disease. *J Natl Cancer Inst* 96: 1577-1584, 2004.

38.   **Kenyon C, Chang J, Gensch E, Rudner A, and Tabtiang R**. A C. elegans mutant that lives twice as long as wild type. *Nature* 366: 461-464, 1993.

39.   **Kinney-Forshee BA, Kinney NE, Steger RW, and Bartke A**. Could a deficiency in growth hormone signaling be beneficial to the aging brain? *Physiol Behav* 80: 589-594, 2004.

40.   **Kolata G**. Steep decline in smoking might be reason for thicker waistlines. In: *Seattle Times*2004, p. Dec. 19.

41.   **Krishnan KJ, Greaves LC, Reeve AK, and Turnbull DM**. Mitochondrial DNA mutations and aging. *Ann N Y Acad Sci* 1100: 227-240, 2007.

42.   **Lam TH, Ho SY, Hedley AJ, Mak KH, and Leung GM**. Leisure time physical activity and mortality in Hong Kong: case-control study of all adult deaths in 1998. *Ann Epidemiol* 14: 391-398, 2004.

43.   **Lee SS, Lee RY, Fraser AG, Kamath RS, Ahringer J, and Ruvkun G**. A systematic RNAi screen identifies a critical role for mitochondria in C. elegans longevity. *Nat Genet* 33: 40-48, 2003.

44. **Li Y, Wang WJ, Cao H, Lu J, Wu C, Hu FY, Guo J, Zhao L, Yang F, Zhang YX, Li W, Zheng GY, Cui H, Chen X, Zhu Z, He H, Dong B, Mo X, Zeng Y, and Tian XL**. Genetic association of FOXO1A and FOXO3A with longevity trait in Han Chinese populations. *Hum Mol Genet* 18: 4897-4904, 2009.

45. **Linford NJ, Schriner SE, and Rabinovitch PS**. Oxidative damage and aging: spotlight on mitochondria. *Cancer Res* 66: 2497-2499, 2006.

46. **Liu L, DiGirolamo CM, Navarro PA, Blasco MA, and Keefe DL**. Telomerase deficiency impairs differentiation of mesenchymal stem cells. *Exp Cell Res* 294: 1-8, 2004.

47. **Lombard DB, Chua KF, Mostoslavsky R, Franco S, Gostissa M, and Alt FW**. DNA repair, genome stability, and aging. *Cell* 120: 497-512, 2005.

48. **Matthews CE, Jurj AL, Shu XO, Li HL, Yang G, Li Q, Gao YT, and Zheng W**. Influence of exercise, walking, cycling, and overall nonexercise physical activity on mortality in Chinese women. *Am J Epidemiol* 165: 1343-1350, 2007.

49. **McClintock D, Gordon LB, and Djabali K**. Hutchinson-Gilford progeria mutant lamin A primarily targets human vascular cells as detected by an anti-Lamin A G608G antibody. *Proc Natl Acad Sci U S A* 103: 2154-2159, 2006.

50. **Moeller SM, Taylor A, Tucker KL, McCullough ML, Chylack LT, Jr., Hankinson SE, Willett WC, and Jacques PF**. Overall adherence to the dietary guidelines for americans is associated with reduced prevalence of early age-related nuclear lens opacities in women. *J Nutr* 134: 1812-1819, 2004.

51. **Novelli V, Viviani Anselmi C, Roncarati R, Guffanti G, Malovini A, Piluso G, and Puca AA**. Lack of replication of genetic associations with human longevity. *Biogerontology* 9: 85-92, 2008.

52. **Ockene IS, and Miller NH**. Cigarette smoking, cardiovascular disease, and stroke: a statement for healthcare professionals from the American Heart Association. American Heart Association Task Force on Risk Reduction. *Circulation* 96: 3243-3247, 1997.

53.   **Orr WC, and Sohal RS**. The effects of catalase gene overexpression on life span and resistance to oxidative stress in transgenic Drosophila melanogaster. *Arch Biochem Biophys* 297: 35-41, 1992.

54.   **Panza F, D'Introno A, Capurso C, Colacicco AM, Seripa D, Pilotto A, Santamato A, Capurso A, and Solfrizzi V**. Lipoproteins, vascular-related genetic factors, and human longevity. *Rejuvenation Res* 10: 441-458, 2007.

55.   **Pawlikowska L, Hu D, Huntsman S, Sung A, Chu C, Chen J, Joyner AH, Schork NJ, Hsueh WC, Reiner AP, Psaty BM, Atzmon G, Barzilai N, Cummings SR, Browner WS, Kwok PY, and Ziv E**. Association of common genetic variation in the insulin/IGF1 signaling pathway with human longevity. *Aging Cell* 8: 460-472, 2009.

56.   **Perez-Rivero G, Ruiz-Torres MP, Rivas-Elena JV, Jerkic M, Diez-Marques ML, Lopez-Novoa JM, Blasco MA, and Rodriguez-Puyol D**. Mice deficient in telomerase activity develop hypertension because of an excess of endothelin production. *Circulation* 114: 309-317, 2006.

57.   **Ramsey KM, Mills KF, Satoh A, and Imai S**. Age-associated loss of Sirt1-mediated enhancement of glucose-stimulated insulin secretion in beta cell-specific Sirt1-overexpressing (BESTO) mice. *Aging Cell* 7: 78-88, 2008.

58.   **Ran Q, Liang H, Ikeno Y, Qi W, Prolla TA, Roberts LJ, 2nd, Wolf N, VanRemmen H, and Richardson A**. Reduction in glutathione peroxidase 4 increases life span through increased sensitivity to apoptosis. *J Gerontol A Biol Sci Med Sci* 62: 932-942, 2007.

59.   **Report**. Dietary Guidelines for Americans edited by HHS,   and   USDA2005,   p. http://www.health.gov/dietaryguidelines/.

60.   **Report**. The Health Consequences of Smoking: A Report of the Surgeon General. edited by Department of Health and Human Services CfDCaP, National Center for Chronic Disease Prevention and Health Promotion, Office on Smoking   and   Health2004,   p. http://www.cdc.gov/tobacco/data_statistics/.

61.   **Report**. Reducing the Health Consequences of Smoking—25 Years of Progress: A Report of the Surgeon General. . edited by HHS, and CDC. Atlanta, GA: 2006, p. http://profiles.nlm.nih.gov/NN/B/B/X/S/.

62.   **Ressler S, Bartkova J, Niederegger H, Bartek J, Scharffetter-Kochanek K, Jansen-Durr P, and Wlaschek M**. p16INK4A is a robust in vivo biomarker of cellular aging in human skin. *Aging Cell* 5: 379-389, 2006.

63.   **Richter T, and von Zglinicki T**. A continuous correlation between oxidative stress and telomere shortening in fibroblasts. *Exp Gerontol* 42: 1039-1042, 2007.

64.   **Ryazanov AG, and Nefsky BS**. Protein turnover plays a key role in aging. *Mech Ageing Dev* 123: 207-213, 2002.

65.   **Sedelnikova OA, Horikawa I, Redon C, Nakamura A, Zimonjic DB, Popescu NC, and Bonner WM**. Delayed kinetics of DNA double-strand break processing in normal and pathological aging. *Aging Cell* 7: 89-100, 2008.

66.   **Sedelnikova OA, Horikawa I, Zimonjic DB, Popescu NC, Bonner WM, and Barrett JC**. Senescing human cells and ageing mice accumulate DNA lesions with unrepairable double-strand breaks. *Nat Cell Biol* 6: 168-170, 2004.

67.   **Selman C, Lingard S, Choudhury AI, Batterham RL, Claret M, Clements M, Ramadani F, Okkenhaug K, Schuster E, Blanc E, Piper MD, Al-Qassab H, Speakman JR, Carmignac D, Robinson IC, Thornton JM, Gems D, Partridge L, and Withers DJ**. Evidence for lifespan extension and delayed age-related biomarkers in insulin receptor substrate 1 null mice. *Faseb J* 22: 807-818, 2008.

68.   **Shringarpure R, and Davies KJ**. Protein turnover by the proteasome in aging and disease. *Free Radic Biol Med* 32: 1084-1089, 2002.

69.   **Sohal RS, and Orr WC**. Relationship between antioxidants, prooxidants, and the aging process. *Ann N Y Acad Sci* 663: 74-84, 1992.

70.   **Suh Y, Atzmon G, Cho MO, Hwang D, Liu B, Leahy DJ, Barzilai N, and Cohen P**. Functionally significant insulin-like growth factor I receptor mutations in centenarians. *Proc Natl Acad Sci U S A* 105: 3438-3442, 2008.

71.   van Heemst D, Beekman M, Mooijaart SP, Heijmans BT, Brandt BW, Zwaan BJ, Slagboom PE, and Westendorp RG. Reduced insulin/IGF-1 signalling and human longevity. *Aging Cell* 4: 79-85, 2005.

72.   **Vaupel JW.** The remarkable improvements in survival at older ages. *Philos Trans R Soc Lond B Biol Sci* 352: 1799-1804, 1997.

73.   **Vaupel JW, Carey JR, Christensen K, Johnson TE, Yashin AI, Holm NV, Iachine IA, Kannisto V, Khazaeli AA, Liedo P, Longo VD, Zeng Y, Manton KG, and Curtsinger JW.** Biodemographic trajectories of longevity. *Science* 280: 855-860, 1998.

74.   **Vaupel JW, and Kistowski VK.** [The remarkable rise in life expectancy and how it will affect medicine]. *Bundesgesundheitsblatt Gesundheitsforschung Gesundheitsschutz* 48: 586-592, 2005.

75.   **Von Zglinicki T.** Replicative senescence and the art of counting. *Exp Gerontol* 38: 1259-1264, 2003.

76.   **von Zglinicki T, Saretzki G, Docke W, and Lotze C.** Mild hyperoxia shortens telomeres and inhibits proliferation of fibroblasts: a model for senescence? *Exp Cell Res* 220: 186-193, 1995.

77.   **Wade N.** New Light Shed on How Enzyme May Play Crucial Role in Cancer. In: *New York Times.* New York: 1995, p. Sept. 5.

78.   **Zahn J, Sonu R, Vogel H, Crane E, Mazan-Mamczarz K, Rabkin R, Davis R, Becker K, Owen A, and Kim S.** Transcriptional profiling of aging in human muscle reveals a common aging signature. *PLoS Genet* 2(7): e115, 2006.

79.   **Zeng Y, Cheng L, Chen H, Cao H, Hauser ER, Liu Y, Xiao Z, Tan Q, Tian XL, and Vaupel JW.** Effects of FOXO genotypes on longevity: a biodemographic analysis. *J Gerontol A Biol Sci Med Sci* 65: 1285-1299, 2010.

80.   **Rose MR, Drapeau MD, Yazdi PG, Shah KH, Moise DB, Thakar RR, Rauser CL, and Mueller LD.** Evolution of late-life mortality in Drosophila melanogaster. *Evolution* 56: 1982-1991, 2002.

81.   **Chen HY, Zajitschek F, and Maklakov AA**. Why ageing stops: heterogeneity explains late-life mortality deceleration in nematodes. *Biol Lett* 9: 20130217, 2013.

82.   **Bartzokis G**. Age-related myelin breakdown: a developmental model of cognitive decline and Alzheimer's disease. *Neurobiol Aging* 25: 5-18; author reply 49-62, 2004.

83.   **Bartzokis G**. Neuroglialpharmacology: myelination as a shared mechanism of action of psychotropic treatments. *Neuropharmacology* 62: 2137-2153, 2012.

84.   **Bartzokis G, Lu PH, and Mintz J**. Quantifying age-related myelin breakdown with MRI: novel therapeutic targets for preventing cognitive decline and Alzheimer's disease. *J Alzheimers Dis* 6: S53-59, 2004.

85.   **Bowley MP, Cabral H, Rosene DL, and Peters A**. Age changes in myelinated nerve fibers of the cingulate bundle and corpus callosum in the rhesus monkey. *J Comp Neurol* 518: 3046-3064, 2010.

86.   **Dickstein DL, Kabaso D, Rocher AB, Luebke JI, Wearne SL, and Hof PR**. Changes in the structural complexity of the aged brain. *Aging Cell* 6: 275-284, 2007.

87.   **Keisala T, Minasyan A, Lou YR, Zou J, Kalueff AV, Pyykko I, and Tuohimaa P**. Premature aging in vitamin D receptor mutant mice. *J Steroid Biochem Mol Biol* 115: 91-97, 2009.

88.   **Tuohimaa P**. Vitamin D and aging. *J Steroid Biochem Mol Biol* 114: 78-84, 2009.

89.   **Tuohimaa P, Keisala T, Minasyan A, Cachat J, and Kalueff A**. Vitamin D, nervous system and aging. *Psychoneuroendocrinology* 34 Suppl 1: S278-286, 2009.

90.   **McCann JC, and Ames BN**. Vitamin K, an example of triage theory: is micronutrient inadequacy linked to diseases of aging? *Am J Clin Nutr* 90: 889-907, 2009.

91.   **Najmi Varzaneh F, Sharifi F, Hossein-Nezhad A, Mirarefin M, Maghbooli Z, Ghaderpanahi M, Larijani B, and Fakhrzadeh H**. Association of vitamin D receptor with longevity and healthy aging. *Acta Med Iran* 51: 236-241, 2013.

92.   **Adrian M, Chanut E, Laurant P, Gaume V, and Berthelot A**. A long-term moderate magnesium-deficient diet

aggravates cardiovascular risks associated with aging and increases mortality in rats. *J Hypertens* 26: 44-52, 2008.

93.   **Barbagallo M, Belvedere M, and Dominguez LJ**. Magnesium homeostasis and aging. *Magnes Res* 22: 235-246, 2009.

94.   **Barbagallo M, and Dominguez LJ**. Magnesium and aging. *Curr Pharm Des* 16: 832-839, 2010.

95.   **Killilea DW, and Maier JA**. A connection between magnesium deficiency and aging: new insights from cellular studies. *Magnes Res* 21: 77-82, 2008.

96.   **McCann JC, and Ames BN**. Adaptive dysfunction of selenoproteins from the perspective of the triage theory: why modest selenium deficiency may increase risk of diseases of aging. *Faseb J* 25: 1793-1814, 2011.

97.   **Ray AL, Semba RD, Walston J, Ferrucci L, Cappola AR, Ricks MO, Xue QL, and Fried LP**. Low serum selenium and total carotenoids predict mortality among older women living in the community: the women's health and aging studies. *J Nutr* 136: 172-176, 2006.

98.   **Semba RD, Ferrucci L, Cappola AR, Ricks MO, Ray AL, Xue QL, Guralnik JM, and Fried LP**. Low Serum Selenium Is Associated with Anemia Among Older Women Living in the Community: the Women's Health and Aging Studies I and II. *Biol Trace Elem Res* 112: 97-107, 2006.

99.   **McColl G, Killilea DW, Hubbard AE, Vantipalli MC, Melov S, and Lithgow GJ**. Pharmacogenetic analysis of lithium-induced delayed aging in Caenorhabditis elegans. *J Biol Chem* 283: 350-357, 2008.

100.   **Tajes M, Yeste-Velasco M, Zhu X, Chou SP, Smith MA, Pallas M, Camins A, and Casadesus G**. Activation of Akt by lithium: pro-survival pathways in aging. *Mech Ageing Dev* 130: 253-261, 2009.

101.   **Zarse K, Terao T, Tian J, Iwata N, Ishii N, and Ristow M**. Low-dose lithium uptake promotes longevity in humans and metazoans. *Eur J Nutr* 50: 387-389, 2011.

102.   **Ayyadevara S, Bharill P, Dandapat A, Hu C, Khaidakov M, Mitra S, Shmookler Reis RJ, and Mehta JL**. Aspirin inhibits oxidant stress, reduces age-associated

functional declines, and extends lifespan of Caenorhabditis elegans. *Antioxid Redox Signal* 18: 481-490, 2013.

103.   **McCowan C, Munro AJ, Donnan PT, and Steele RJ**. Use of aspirin post-diagnosis in a cohort of patients with colorectal cancer and its association with all-cause and colorectal cancer specific mortality. *Eur J Cancer* 49: 1049-1057, 2013.

104.   **Rothwell PM**. Aspirin in prevention of sporadic colorectal cancer: current clinical evidence and overall balance of risks and benefits. *Recent Results Cancer Res* 191: 121-142, 2013.

105.   **Sutcliffe P, Connock M, Gurung T, Freeman K, Johnson S, Kandala NB, Grove A, Gurung B, Morrow S, and Clarke A**. Aspirin for prophylactic use in the primary prevention of cardiovascular disease and cancer: a systematic review and overview of reviews. *Health Technol Assess* 17: 1-253, 2013.

106.   **Wang JQ, Wu GR, Wang Z, Dai XP, and Li XR**. Long-term Clinical Outcomes of Statin Use for Chronic Heart Failure: A Meta-analysis of 15 Prospective Studies. *Heart Lung Circ* 2013.

107.   **Blasco MA, Funk W, Villeponteau B, and Greider CW**. Functional characterization and developmental regulation of mouse telomerase RNA. *Science* 269: 1267-1270, 1995.

108.   **Feng J, Funk WD, Wang SS, Weinrich SL, Avilion AA, Chiu CP, Adams RR, Chang E, Allsopp RC, Yu J, Andrews WH, Greider CW, and Villeponteau B**. The RNA component of human telomerase. *Science* 269: 1236-1241, 1995.

109.   **Harley CB, and Villeponteau B**. Telomeres and telomerase in aging and cancer. *Curr Opin Genet Dev* 5: 249-255, 1995.

110.   **Linskens MH, Feng J, Andrews WH, Enlow BE, Saati SM, Tonkin LA, Funk WD, and Villeponteau B**. Cataloging altered gene expression in young and senescent cells using enhanced differential display. *Nucleic Acids Res* 23: 3244-3251, 1995.

111.   **Matsagas K, Lim DB, Horwitz M, Rizza CL, Mueller LD, Villeponteau B, and Rose MR**. Long-term functional side-effects of stimulants and sedatives in Drosophila melanogaster. *PLoS One* 4: e6578, 2009.

112.   **Villeponteau B**. The heterochromatin loss model of aging. *Exp Gerontol* 32: 383-394, 1997.

113.   **Jones OR, Scheuerlein A, Salguero-Gomez R, Camarda CG, Schaible R, Casper BB, Dahlgren JP, Ehrlen J, Garcia MB, Menges ES, Quintana-Ascencio PF, Caswell H, Baudisch A, and Vaupel JW**. Diversity of ageing across the tree of life. *Nature Published online on Dec. 8,* 2013.

Made in the USA
Charleston, SC
10 May 2014